The Coming Revolution in Medicine

The MIT Press
Massachusetts Institute of Technology
Cambridge, Massachusetts, and London, England

The
Coming
Revolution
in
Medicine
David D. Rutstein

To Ruthie
for
Peace and Happiness

Foreword

Everyone who has had the ill fortune to be a patient in one of today's hospitals—be it part of a major medical center or a small county institution—has witnessed first-hand the complexities of modern surgery, diagnosis, and care of the sick. Surgeons, general practitioners, nurses, and orderlies all operate within confusing and often contradictory job categories. Most of them are already overworked, and as Medicare releases the expectations of the general public for better health care, their problems will increase.

Dr. Rutstein's four essays, which are based on a series of lectures that he delivered at the Massachusetts Institute of Technology in the fall of 1966, provide a thoughtful and provocative analysis of the present crisis in medicine. They mark the author as a bold and vigorous leader in today's revolution in medical research, education, and care.

As Dr. Rutstein so forcefully points out, the answer will not come merely from finding more doctors or more nurses but, rather, can come only from a comprehensive systems review of the whole domain of health care leading to the interweaving of new skills, new technology, and new managerial methodologies into the total fabric. It will call for the building of new paths for the exchange of knowledge between the life scientist, the physical scientist, the doctor, the engineer, and the institutional administrator.

For several years now, the faculty at M.I.T. has been searching for these paths. It realizes only too well that it is facing more than problems of vocabulary or of semantics. It is seeking common denominators for the foundations upon which to build new structures of knowledge and skills. The activities of the Faculty Committee on Engineering and Living Systems—formed about three years ago within the School of Engineering —are steps in this direction. The degree to which its actions uncovered a deep and vigorous interest among both faculty and students in problems of medical science and practice was most heartening. The invitation to Dr. Rutstein to give his series of four lectures sprang from the activity of this committee and serves as one more link in the new structures that have been emerging as our faculty continue to strengthen the friendly and cooperative relations between M.I.T. and its neighboring medical schools.

As Head of the Department of Preventive Medicine at Harvard since its establishment in 1947 and as a qualified specialist in internal medicine and cardiology, Dr. Rutstein has influenced students and faculty to integrate preventive concepts with actual care of patients. He has instituted as part of his teaching an assessment by students of the medical care afforded by specific communities, selected by the students themselves, leading to the crucial question, "How can we do away with unnecessary disease, disability, or untimely death by utilizing existing resources—both medical and technological—more effectively?"

With this personal involvement in the teaching and learning process and with a background of three years as Deputy Commissioner and Director of Laboratories of the New York City Department of Health under Mayor Fiorello La Guardia, who else but Dr. Rutstein could be better qualified to speak out on such a crucial topic at this time?

GORDON S. BROWN
Dean of the School of Engineering
Massachusetts Institute of Technology

Cambridge, Massachusetts
June 1, 1967

Contents

Introduction

These essays on *The Coming Revolution in Medicine* are based on a series of four lectures delivered at the Massachusetts Institute of Technology in the late fall of 1966. They comprise writings, begun in the 1950's, concerned with an examination of the current medical scene and a look into the future. These explorations included an evaluation of the rapidly developing relationship of mathematics, the physical and engineering sciences, and technology to biology and medicine.

The future role of the general physician was surveyed for the lay reader in "Do You Really Want a Family Doctor?" in *Harper's Magazine* and later in the professional medical journal, *The Lancet*. The need for objective standards in medicine and in medical care was documented in a lecture to the College of Physicians of Philadelphia. The widening spectrum of career opportunities in medicine was defined in the Class Day Address of 1962 at the Harvard Medical School. The framework for regionalization of medical care services was detailed in the Lowell Lecture of 1963, and the potential impact of Medicare was estimated in "Reflections on the Medicine of the Future" at the 1965 New York Academy of Medicine Health Conference.

At the same time, I explored the growing program relating mathematics, engineering, the physical sciences, and technology at the Massachusetts Institute of Technology with medicine and medical and biological research at the Harvard Medical School. These latter activities were initiated by a conversation in Poland which I had in 1959 with Dr. Antoni Horst, then Dean of the Medical School of Poznan, who urged me to take advantage of the great opportunities in Boston and to explore the possibility of "bringing mathematics into medicine."

A conference later that year with Professor Jerome Wiesner, then Director of the Research Laboratory of Electronics, Professor Gordon Brown, Dean of the School of Engineering, and Professor Walter Rosenblith at the Massachusetts Institute of Technology resulted in a joint program between the Department of Preventive Medicine and the Massachusetts Institute of Technology conducted by Professor Murray Eden. It began by providing consultation in biomathematics to the faculty at the Harvard Medical School. During the following year, a program on mathematics and the medical sciences was presented by experts in the field to the Harvard medical faculty. In 1960, a teaching program for Harvard Medical School undergraduates was initiated in biomathematics, and is now included in the curriculum. Later, I elaborated these ideas in a guest lecture on "Mathematics and Computers in Medicine of the Future" at the Annual Meeting of the British Medical Association in Manchester, England, in 1964. I put all this information together for the first time early in 1966 in lectures delivered at the Swedish Medical Society and at medical schools in Uppsala, Stockholm, Göteborg, and Malmö-Lund.

In this book, I survey the present chaotic medical scene and make an assessment of the needs and resources of American medicine with an eye toward a systematic plan for the future. I begin by examining some of the reasons for the widespread disquietude resulting from "The Paradox of Modern Medicine." This paradox is the seeming contradiction of our mushrooming medical research program and the slowdown in the improvement of our national health. In the first essay, I document this paradox and explore the nature of the forces responsible for its existence.

Next, in "The Tangled Web of Medical Care," I am concerned with the primitive nature of our unplanned medical care system — so well characterized by Professor Harvey Brooks' trenchant remark, "Medicine is a cottage industry." In evolving a more systematic approach to medical care, the possible contributions of the Massachusetts Institute of Technology loomed large. As Professor Rosenblith and I explored this possibility, we identified four separate, relevant, active interfaces between schools of technology and medicine. The first interface is concerned with the application of systems analysis and operations research in the management and control of such complex systems as a hospital, a medical care plan, or a research program.

The third essay, "The Impact of Contemporary Technology and Automation," may be brought into focus by the second, third, and fourth interfaces between technology and medicine. The second interface comprises the development of machines, physically attached to and immediately concerned with the life or health of the patient, whether in the form of an artificial organ such as the kidney or heart, a feedback (servo) mechanism to control blood pressure or other human physiologic functions, an electronic prosthesis to help paraplegic patients to walk, or a sensory aid to help the blind to read.

The third interface describes the application of automation to such medical situations as laboratory testing of the chemical assay of sugar in the blood and the counting of blood cells; scanning machinery for the reading of electrocardiograms and other electronic records; analytic instrumentation to aid the physician in medical diagnosis; or helping a nurse to monitor seriously ill patients in the hospital's intensive-care or emergency unit.

The fourth interface — the most important of all — is concerned with research to yield new knowledge in the physical and engineering sciences and with the development of new mathematical theory, all relevant to the solution of biological and medical problems. Now that the morphological and the biochemical sciences have become an integral part of medical education, research, and care, it is time to overcome the lag in the application of the physical sciences and of mathematics to medicine. We are concerned at this fourth interface with fundamental research, in contrast with the application of existing knowledge in the first three interfaces. At every interface, the computer is an essential working tool.

The first three analytical essays provide the background for an understanding of "A Plan for the Medicine of the Future," the subject of the fourth essay. That plan will propose not a Utopian solution but a series of guidelines and studies to eliminate some of the major obstacles to the improvement of our national health.

A series of essays can outline only in skeleton fashion the nature of the problems and the lines along which progress may be made. As this small volume goes to press and as I watch reactions to it I am beginning to write a more detailed book on the medicine of the future to flesh out the bones put together here.

One word of caution. Many medical plans have as their sole objective the efficient use of medical personnel, institutions, and financial and other resources. My plan does not have that limited objective. It is not enough to study the machinery of a program. We hear a great deal about relative costs, the availability of beds, use of laboratory services, the required number of physicians and paramedical and ancillary personnel, and the size of budgets. But these measures do not really evaluate effectiveness. In the final analysis, the effectiveness of a health program must be measured by a decrease in disease, disability, or untimely death, or the program is of no practical use. The laboratories, the men in the white suits, the budgets, are all parts of the machine and, of course, must be brought together in an effective way. But we must not become so interested in the machine itself that we forget what it was made to do — to keep people well.

I do not mean to belittle the kinds of measurements that tell us what percentage of the time a hospital bed is occupied or the most effective method of payment of hospital costs. These are extremely important questions from the economic point of view. But for the effectiveness of a program, we need professional measuring sticks or standards, based on the state at the particular time of medical science and technology. Reliable methods of measurement are being developed to measure the efficiency of the medical care machine in terms of human betterment.

It is appropriate that I make clear what I have not attempted to do in this book. This book is not a blueprint for a medical care plan of the future. Rather, I have projected lines along which progress may be made and suggested the kinds of studies that could yield a better definition of future trends.

I make a conscious attempt not to focus this book on the economic problems of medicine. Instead, I have indicated how medical care and health programs must be based on the sum of our scientific knowledge and optimal professional skills and institutional, technical, and social resources, and then scaled down under the pressures of economic and other limitations. Too long have medical care programs been initiated and planned mainly about economic resources, under the assumption that the highest quality of medical care will automatically be provided. My plan approaches the problem from the opposite direction, that of the highest quality of medical care that might be provided if we could make available all existing knowledge, skills, and optimal resources.

Finally, I would hope that this book would precipitate an active, thorough, and informed discussion so that we could join together in developing a plan that would have beneficial effects on our national health.

Obviously, many colleagues and friends within and without the medical profession have contributed ideas, thoughts, and discussions that have helped to clarify my thinking. Unfortunately, I can acknowledge only those who have been of immediate help in the actual writing of this book. I am indebted to Provost Jerome Wiesner, Dean Gordon Brown, and Professor Walter Rosenblith of the Massachusetts Institute of Technology for their patient attempts to educate me about relevant physical and engineering sciences, mathematics, and technology.

I am particularly appreciative of the thoughtful criticisms and suggestions following careful review of this manuscript by Sir Theodore Fox, Editor Emeritus of *The Lancet*, Dr. Robert H. Ebert, Dean of the Harvard Medical School, Dean Harvey Brooks, Department of

Engineering and Applied Physics at Harvard University, Dr. Alexander Leaf, Jackson Professor of Medicine at the Harvard Medical School, Dr. Jack Masur, Director of the Clinical Center of the National Institutes of Health, Dr. Nathalie Masse of the International Children's Center in Paris, and Dr. Robert Burden, of the Faculty of Public Health, and of the Division of Engineering and Applied Physics at Harvard University.

Dr. Osler L. Peterson, Rita J. Nickerson, and other members of the staff of the Department of Preventive Medicine have contributed research data and time and effort to the manifold tasks in the production of this book. Special acknowledgment must be made to Patricia W. Eden for her constructive and firm editorial assistance. I also wish to thank Alfred Popoli for administrative help and Ernestine Macedo for typing the material.

I am grateful to the Commonwealth Fund for their generous grant providing administrative, editorial and library assistance, secretarial support, and travel funds, which have lightened my administrative responsibilities and released my time for the preparation of these essays, and to the American Academy of Arts and Sciences for making available in the summer of 1966 pleasant, serene surroundings in which to work. Finally, I appreciate the opportunity provided by the Massachusetts Institute of Technology for the presentation of these lectures.

DAVID D. RUTSTEIN, M.D.

April 25, 1967

The Paradox of Modern Medicine

During the past half century, we have made great health progress. Indeed, the trends of modern medicine are breathtaking. Medical science has learned how to change the course of the natural history of disease, to alleviate suffering, to terminate severe illness, to prevent crippling, and to postpone untimely death. Progress has been favored by an increasing standard of living, better housing, and a broader base of education. Wonder drugs like penicillin now provide immediate cure for diseases such as lobar pneumonia, which two decades ago claimed one quarter of its victims. As a result, there has been a decrease in infant mortality and a concomitant increase in life expectancy. Many individuals have been spared the great burden of such chronic illnesses as tuberculosis. Many major fatal diseases such as whooping cough, poliomyelitis, diphtheria, and typhoid fever have been prevented. But, as we shall see, there has been for almost two decades a steady leveling off in our health progress. Curiously this change in trend has coincided with an enormous expansion in our national medical research program.

Mushrooming of Medical Science

The unprecedented expansion in medical research in the United States is documented at every turn. Whether we look at the expenditure of medical research funds, the expansion of laboratory facilities, the number and proportion of physicians and preclinical scientists occupied with medical research, or the number of medical journals and published scientific articles, the trend is sharply upward.

The most striking example of this mushrooming is the growth of federal expenditures for medical research. Thirty years ago, in 1937, the budget of the National Institutes of Health included less than $150 thousand for the subsidy of biomedical research projects in universities and hospitals. Twenty years ago, it rose to less than $1 million, with almost nothing for research fellowships, training grants, or construction of research facilities.

In 1965, the National Institutes of Health distributed more than $1 billion to universities, hospitals, and health agencies in support of biomedical research. This included substantial amounts for research fellowships, training programs for research, equipment, and the construction of laboratories and clinical investigation facilities. To these expenditures must also be added the growing cost of the intramural research program of the NIH which in thirty years has risen from one third of $1 million to about $90 million. In spite of the dire predictions that such an increase in federal expenditures for medical research would cause voluntary contributions and industrial support to drop off sharply, this has not happened. The nonfederal support of biomedical research has increased about tenfold since World War II.

There is no need to elaborate many details of the growth of research facilities and personnel. If one examines the product of the medical scientific establishment, the increase is phenomenal. The American Medical Association in 1958, the last year in which it published the *Quarterly Cumulative Index Medicus,* indexed 60,000 articles. For 1964, it is estimated that 220,000 medical articles were published in more than 13,000 journals throughout the world. This enormous expansion in our national medical research program together with our lagging national health picture is the paradox of modern medicine.

Our Health Indices

Let us take a look at the indices of health to see what our national progress has been. Our most valid indices are life expectancy and infant mortality. Life expectancy at birth is a theoretical estimate in a particular year of the average length of life of a newborn baby.[1] Life expectancy is an expression of the burden imposed upon us by all fatal illnesses throughout our entire lifetime.

The second index, the infant mortality rate, is the

[1] Life expectancy of a newborn baby in a particular year is calculated on the assumption that he would be exposed throughout his lifetime to the age-specific mortality rates for that year.

number of infants who die in their first year of life out of every thousand who are born alive. Infant mortality is a sensitive indicator of the effectiveness of medicine in the social structure and of the guidance provided to the public by the medical profession. This rate can be directly affected by changing living and sanitation standards, by better maternal and obstetrical care, by adequate nutrition, and by more careful pediatric supervision and medical care during the first year of life. In a sense, this index is an expression of what a society under the guidance of its physicians will do for its mothers and babies.

These indices have the limitations that they are concerned only with mortality and provide no measures of nonfatal illness. Unfortunately, we do not yet have comparable international indices to measure the relative impact of illness. In the United States we are just beginning to collect precise information about the amount and distribution of illness, that is, morbidity, as distinct from mortality. The National Center for Health Statistics of the United States Public Health Service established the National Health Survey in 1958, which now supplies us with current information on the state of our national health. As data on illness and disability are collected and analyzed in many countries, we shall develop international indices of illness to supplement those of life expectancy and infant mortality. We shall then have a more thoroughgoing and up-to-date picture of our national health as illness and death wax and wane.

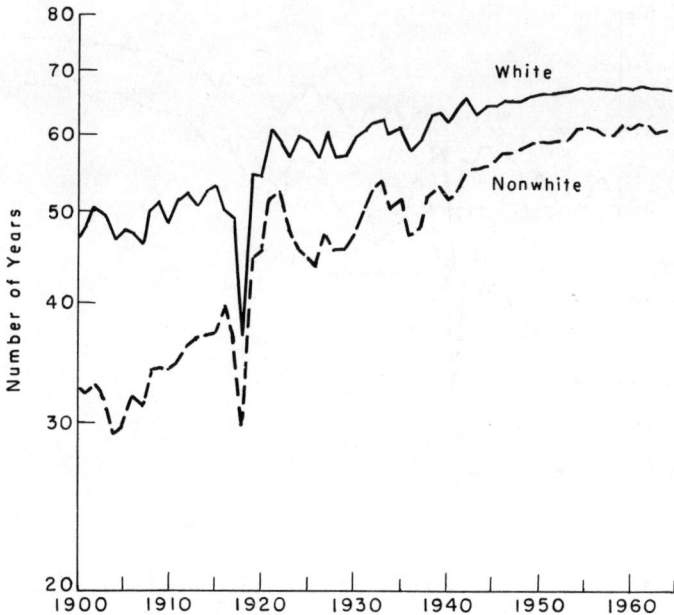

Figure 1.   Expectation of life at birth in the United States, 1900–1964: Males.
(Data include all states after 1933.)

Nevertheless, our mortality indices do yield useful information. Life expectancy of both white and nonwhite males and females has gradually increased in the United States during the last half century (see Figures 1 and 2)[2] as the health status of our country has improved.

[2] The sharp drop for both male and female life expectancy between 1918 and 1920 resulted from the great influenza pandemic at that time. We tend to forget what a serious impact that epidemic had on the health of our country.

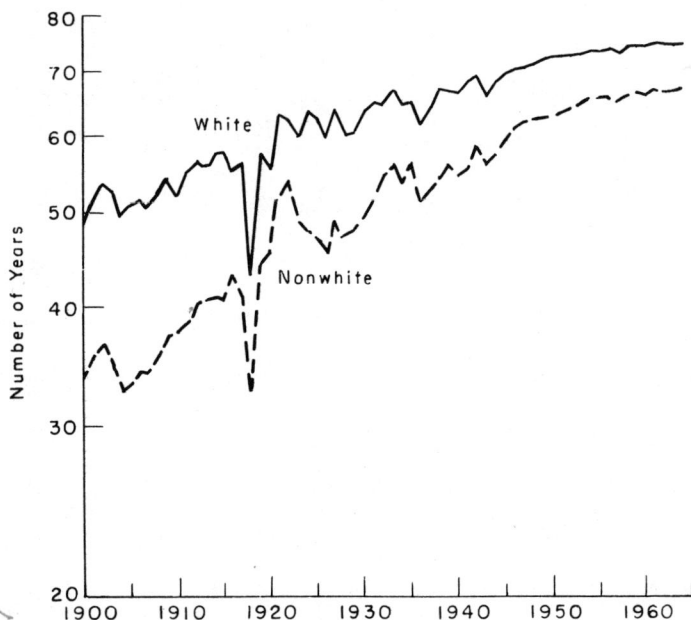

Figure 2.   Expectation of life at birth in the United States,
1900–1964: Females.
(Data include all states after 1933.)

But in these same charts we begin to see warning
signals. During the past two decades, the lengthening of
life expectancy has ground almost to a halt. Indeed, we
have failed to keep up with the improved life expectancy
in many other countries, and the trend has worsened in
the last several years. Let us compare United Nations
statistics compiled in the years 1959 and 1966.[3] During

[3] Actually, for the United States, life expectancies are those of
1958 and 1963 — an interval of five years (Tables 1 and 2).

this interval, the life expectancy of males in the United States dropped from thirteenth to twenty-second place (see Table 1) and female life expectancy from seventh to tenth place among the countries of the world (see Table 2). Thus, during that seven-year interval, while life expectancy was increasing slowly in the United States, improvement was more rapid in nine other countries for males and in three other countries for females.

This same lag in health improvement has been demon-

Table 1. Expectation of Life at Birth: Males

1959*

Country	Latest Year Reported	Years of Life
Norway	1951–55	71.11
Netherlands	1953–55	71.0
Sweden	1957	70.82
Israel		
(*Jewish population*)	1959	70.23
Denmark	1951–55	69.87
New Zealand		
(*European population*)	1950–52	68.29
England and Wales	1959	68.1
Canada	1955–57	67.61
Northern Ireland	1957–59	67.44
Czechoslovakia	1958	67.23
Australia	1953–55	67.14
West Germany	1958–59	66.67
UNITED STATES	1958	66.4

* Year of Tabulation.

Table 1. (Continued)

1965*

Country	Latest Year Reported	Years of Life
Netherlands	1956–60	71.4
Sweden	1962	71.3
Norway	1951–55	71.1
Israel		
(*Jewish population*)	1963	70.9
Iceland	1951–60	70.7
Denmark	1956–60	70.4
Switzerland	1959–61	69.5
Canada	1960–62	68.4
New Zealand		
(*European population*)	1955–57	68.2
England and Wales	1961–63	68.0
Northern Ireland	1961–63	67.6
Greece	1960–62	67.5
Eastern Germany	1960–61	67.3
Spain	1960	67.3
Czechoslovakia	1962	67.2
France	1963	67.2
Japan	1963	67.2
Australia	1953–55	67.1
Puerto Rico	1959–61	67.1
Malta	1961–63	67.0
West Germany	1960–62	66.9
UNITED STATES	1963	66.6

* Year of Tabulation.

Table 2. Expectation of Life at Birth: Females

1959*

Country	Latest Year Reported	Years of Life
Norway	1951–55	74.70
Sweden	1957	74.29
Netherlands	1953–55	73.9
England and Wales	1959	73.8
Canada	1955	72.92
Australia	1953–55	72.75
UNITED STATES	1958	72.7

1965*

Country	Latest Year Reported	Years of Life
Sweden	1962	75.4
Iceland	1951–60	75.0
Netherlands	1956–60	74.8
Switzerland	1959–61	74.8
Norway	1951–55	74.7
Canada	1960–62	74.2
France	1963	74.1
England and Wales	1961–63	73.9
Denmark	1956–60	73.8
UNITED STATES	1963	73.4

* Year of Tabulation.

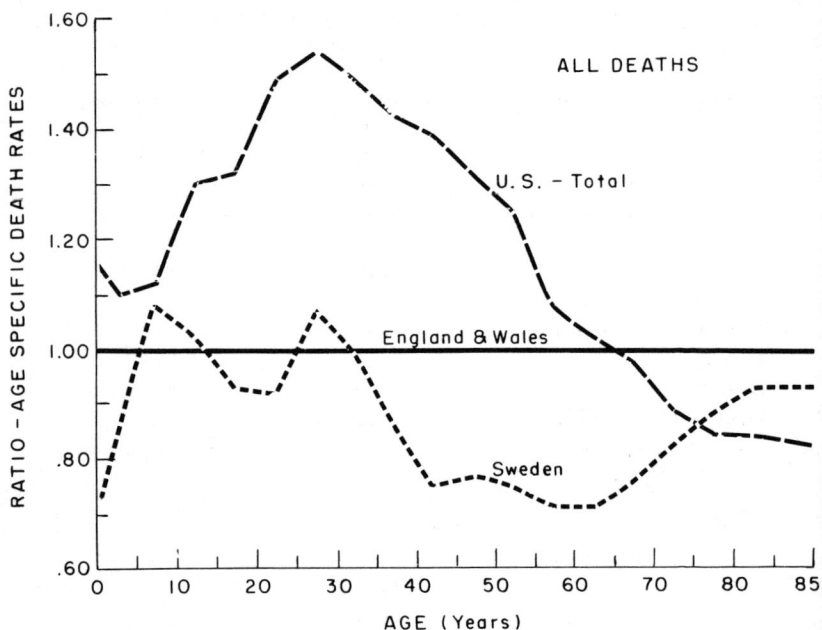

Figure 3.   Ratio of age-specific death rates in the
United States and Sweden to England and Wales.
(*All deaths 1961.*)

strated by a recent comparative study in the Department
of Preventive Medicine at the Harvard Medical School [4]
of death rates in Sweden, England and Wales, and the
United States (see Figure 3). If the death rates in each

[4] Alex M. Burgess, Jr., Theodore Colton, and Osler L. Peterson, "Categorical Programs for Heart Disease, Cancer and Stroke, Lessons from International Death-Rate Comparisons," *The New England Journal of Medicine*, 273 (September 2, 1965), 533–537.

decade for England and Wales are plotted as a straight line, it is clear from the curve for the United States that the latter's death rates in each decade up to age 60 are consistently higher than those for either of the two other countries.

It is interesting that in the "middle years of life" (ages 15–44), the death rates in the United States are higher than those in Sweden for every major grouping of causes of death except one (Table 3). Actually, some causes are strikingly higher; for example, cirrhosis of the liver and hypertension are five to ten times higher in the United States than they are in Sweden. The only exception is suicide, which is one and a quarter times higher in Sweden than in the United States. But we more than make up for this slight advantage in suicide rates with our excessive homicide rates: nine times as high for women, and seventeen times as high for men.

All in all, as far as life expectancy is concerned, we are not doing very well. There is much room for improvement.

Now let us look at the most sensitive index — infant mortality. We have seen a marvelous improvement in infant survival in the last half century. In 1915, about 100 of every 1,000 babies born alive died before they reached their first birthday. Now fewer than 25 die in their first year of life in the United States.

But once again the warning signals are flying. During

Table 3. *Age-Adjusted Death Rates per 100,000 Population, and Ratios of United States to Swedish Death Rates 1961*

Cause of Death	Death Rate for Males 15–44 Years of Age		Ratio of United States to Sweden for Males 15–44 Years of Age	Death Rate for Females 15–44 Years of Age		Ratio of United States to Sweden for Females 15–44 Years of Age
	United States	Sweden		United States	Sweden	
Infectious and parasitic diseases	4.5	3.5	1.3	3.8	2.5	1.5
Malignant tumors	25.7	21.8	1.2	32.5	26.8	1.2
Strokes	7.1	4.6	1.5	7.1	4.2	1.7
Rheumatic heart disease	5.2	1.8	2.9	5.3	2.3	2.3
Arteriosclerotic and degenerative heart disease	34.5	8.4	4.1	7.2	1.3	5.5
Hypertension, with and without heart disease	3.9	0.8	4.9	3.5	0.5	7.0
Influenza, pneumonia, and bronchitis	5.3	2.4	2.2	3.6	1.7	2.1
Cirrhosis of liver	6.2	1.2	5.2	4.4	0.6	7.3
Complications of childbirth	—	—	—	4.2	1.4	3.0
Other diseases	38.5	28.0	1.4	31.3	22.3	1.4
TOTAL (nonexternal)	130.9	72.5	1.8	102.9	63.7	1.6
Motor-vehicle accidents	43.2	21.8	2.0	11.2	5.1	2.2
Other accidents	31.8	25.3	1.3	6.1	2.1	1.6
Suicide	14.6	19.3	0.8	5.3	7.5	0.7
Homicide	11.9	0.7	17.0	3.8	0.4	9.5
TOTAL (external)	101.5	67.1	1.5	26.4	15.1	1.7
TOTAL (all causes)	232.4	139.6	1.7	129.3	78.8	1.6

the past two or three decades, as first pointed out by Moryiama,[5] the improvement in our infant mortality rate has slowed down. Actually, if we look carefully at

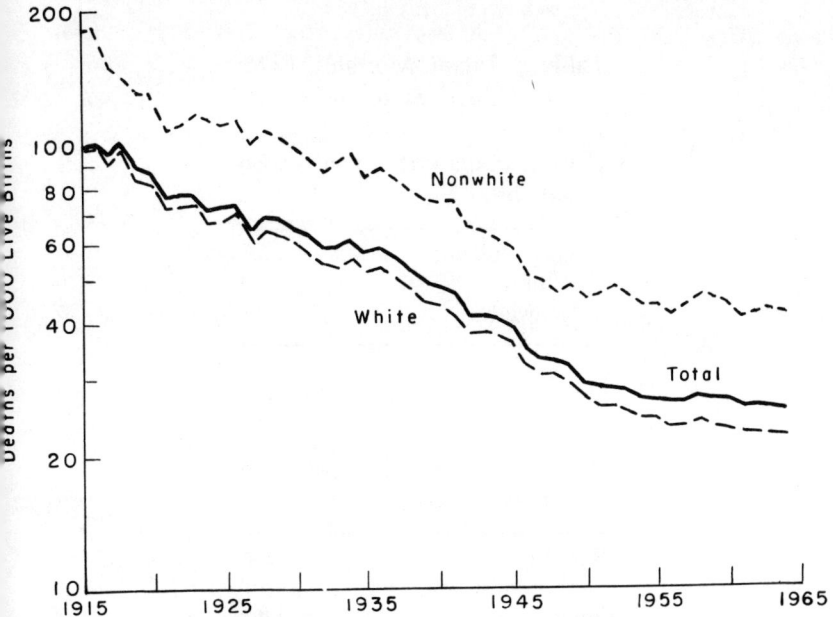

Figure 4.   Infant mortality rates in the United States, 1915–1964.
(Data include all states after 1933.)

Figure 4 we see a most ominous sign. We had always hoped that with the advances of modern medicine and the bubbling affluence of our democratic society the

[5] I. M. Moriyama, "Recent Change in Infant Mortality Trend," *Public Health Reports*, 75 (May 1960), 391–405.

higher death rate among nonwhite infants would come down to the lower level of the white population. But exactly the opposite has been the case. The nonwhite rate (41.1) is now (see Table 4) twice as high as the

Table 4. Infant Mortality Rates in the United States by Color, 1964
(Deaths under one year per 1,000 infants born alive)

Total population	24.8
White	21.6
Nonwhite	41.1

Table 5. Infant Mortality Rates, 1959
(Deaths under one year per 1,000 infants born alive)

Sweden	16.6
Netherlands	16.8
Norway	18.7
New Zealand (*excluding Maoris*)	19.9
Australia	21.5
England and Wales	22.2
Switzerland	22.2
Denmark	22.5
Finland	23.6
Czechoslovakia	25.8
UNITED STATES	26.4

white rate (21.6). This discrepancy in infant death rates between the races is increasing year by year.

This recent slowdown in infant survival is reflected in our international standing. In 1959, we stood eleventh among the countries of the world (Table 5), and that is bad enough. With our lagging improvement during the interval from 1959 to 1965 (Table 6), seven other coun-

Table 6. Infant Mortality Rates, 1965
(Deaths under one year per 1,000 infants born alive)

Sweden	14.2*
Netherlands	14.4
Norway	16.8*
Finland	17.4
Switzerland	17.7
Denmark	18.7
England and Wales	19.0
Australia	19.1*
New Zealand	19.5
Japan	20.4*
Czechoslovakia	21.2*
France	22.1
Israel (Jewish population)	22.7
Scotland	23.1
West Germany	23.9
Belgium	24.0
Canada	24.7*
UNITED STATES	24.8

* Rate for 1964.

tries, including France, Japan, Belgium, and Canada, have passed us, and we are now eighteenth from the top of the list.

The slowdown has another curious aspect. If we examine the infant mortality rates individually for each of the states of the Union, we find in most of them that their present rate is about where it was in the late 1940's, regardless of how high or low it was at that time. For instance, the State of Massachusetts leveled off just below 20, while Mississippi stabilized at a rate of about 40 infant deaths per 1,000 live births (Figure 5). Obviously, the doubled rate of Mississippi is due at least in part to the high nonwhite infant mortality rate and the large Negro population. This dismal fact does not justify the Mississippi infant death rate nor our high national rate. On the contrary, it is further documentation that we are not doing our best, that the paradox of modern medicine in our country is real, and that it has a greater impact on our nonwhite population.

But let us not be misled. Our poor showing in infant mortality is not due entirely to our high nonwhite infant mortality rates. Too many white babies are also dying in the United States. Among our fifty states, Utah in 1962 had the lowest white infant mortality rate (19.8). In that same year the province of Örebro in Sweden had the highest infant mortality rate (19.8) of all of the provinces in Sweden — exactly the same as in Utah. Thus, forty-nine states of our Union had a higher white

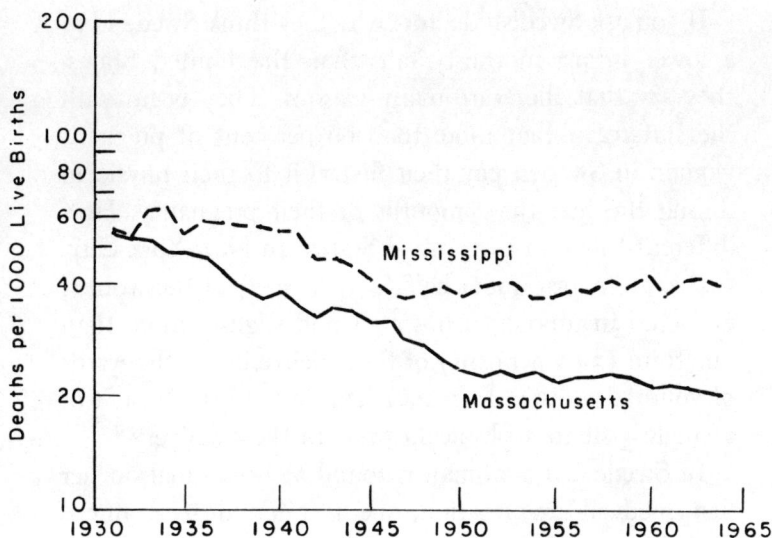

Figure 5.   Infant mortality rates for Massachusetts
and Mississippi, 1930–1964.

infant mortality rate than the highest provincial rate in
Sweden.

I should like to make the firm statement at this time
that the differences in infant mortality rates between
Sweden, other Western countries, and the United States
are real ones. Sweden and the United States use the same
World Health Organization criteria for the definition of
a live birth. I have myself examined the use of this definition in Sweden and I believe that the Swedes can count
dead babies as accurately as we can.

If you ask Swedish doctors why they think Sweden has a lower infant mortality rate than the United States, they say that there are many reasons. They begin with the statement that more than 90 per cent of pregnant women in Sweden pay their first visit to their physician during the first three months of their pregnancy. How different this is in the United States: In New York City, for example, just under half (47 per cent) of the women delivered in municipal hospitals and slightly more than one third (34.5 per cent) of those delivered on the wards of voluntary hospitals in 1961 had not had the benefit of a single visit to a physician prior to their delivery.[6]

In Sweden, if a woman is found to be normal on her first medical examination, she is referred to a nurse-midwife who follows her closely throughout her pregnancy. The midwife must report any serious event in the pregnancy to the patient's physician — otherwise, she may lose her license. The nurse-midwife works closely with the patient throughout her pregnancy, visits her home, and keeps a close watch for warning signals. The physician in Sweden with the assistance of the midwife can follow his patient more closely than can the unaided physician in the United States.

At term, if the pregnancy has been normal, the nurse-

[6] These figures are published by the Maternity Center Association of New York City and have been printed in the *Journal of the American Medical Association*, 187 (January 11, 1964), 35–38.

midwife, working under the supervision of the physician, is in attendance on the patient from the moment she arrives in labor until after she is delivered. In contrast, when one walks into the labor room of an American hospital one finds the inexperienced husband rather than the trained midwife holding the hand of the patient.

The ability of the nurse-midwife to perform normal deliveries makes it unnecessary to schedule deliveries in Sweden as busy American physicians are often forced to do. As a result, in normal deliveries in Sweden, membranes are rarely ruptured, drugs to induce labor are infrequently prescribed, instruments are less commonly used, and there are fewer surgical interventions. The Swedish physicians then conclude — in the light of these facts, that it is not surprising for Sweden to have a lower infant mortality rate than the United States.

Instead of spending our time in fruitless argument as to the validity of the international statistics on infant mortality we would do better to direct our efforts toward saving the lives of American babies. It is clear that in certain parts of our country, in the jungles of our large cities, and for our nonwhite populations, infant mortality rates are extraordinarily high. Fortunately, organizations such as the Massachusetts Medical Society have recognized the serious nature of this problem and have begun intensive studies on infant mortality in order to identify the preventable deaths. With such information, an open mind, and an active program, we can look forward in the future to the saving of the lives of many babies in the United States.

The Paradox in the Framework of Medical Practice

We have seen that there is a sharp discrepancy between the rapid mushrooming of medical science and the slowing improvement in the health of our country. The paradox is a real one.

We must now ask ourselves whether the paradox can be resolved within the present framework of medical practice. Our pattern of medical care has been with us for more than half a century, has worked well in its time, and has assumed an air of permanence. The physician has been practicing in relative isolation in his home or in a professional building. The hospital has been going its self-centered way, adding beds or facilities at the behest of its staff or at the urging of a trustee. Local health departments, by imposed tradition, have been kept out of the hospital and have been safely isolated in city hall from becoming involved with medical care. Too many people have been receiving their care in inadequate clinics through the charity of the individual physician or from a welfare doctor. The large teaching hospital affiliated with the medical school has been giving high-quality inpatient care for diseases of interest to its staff while showing little or no concern for the continuity of medical care for the patient before his admission and after his discharge from the hospital. The medical school has been going ahead blindly with its fixed curriculum that is guaranteed to provide the basic education for whatever career the future physician may decide to follow.

For those opposed to change, the picture of our present medical system is a comfortable one to be maintained at all costs. But the old edifice is beginning to crumble. More physicians are now working full time in medical schools, in industry, and in government, and many fewer are in private practice. Community demands on the hospitals are beginning to make themselves felt. The artificial line between preventive and curative medicine is being obliterated, as demonstrated by the recent appointments of a single commissioner for joint departments of health and hospitals in such cities as New York and Boston. Labor plans and prepayment programs are covering an increasing proportion of the costs of medical care for employed low-income groups. New federal programs require cooperative health planning, which in turn will force reluctant state health departments into medical care activities. Medicare has taken the treatment of the aged out of the charity framework. Some medical schools and their teaching hospitals are becoming actively concerned about the quality of medical care in their communities.

But much more is needed. As we examine the pressures that have brought us to our present state, it will become clear that our national health status will not be markedly improved and the basic paradox will not be eliminated if we do not make significant changes in the present framework of medical practice.

The Pressures Behind the Paradox

The pressures that have brought American medicine to its present paradox include the explosion of scientific knowledge, the trend toward specialization, spiraling costs, changing public expectations, and burgeoning changes in the structure of our society with its accelerating depersonalization. Relatively little can be done to eliminate the pressures. Our task is to harness them to advantage so that they will force improvement in medical care.

The Explosion of Medical Knowledge

An explosion of knowledge has taken place in medicine just as it has in all scientific fields. The conscientious physician is staggered by the rapidity with which changes are taking place so that it becomes more and more difficult for him to introduce them into his practice. In his harried moments, he wishes that science would take a vacation so that he could catch up with what has already been discovered. At the next moment, when he is frustrated by diseases of unknown cause and the serious illnesses that he cannot treat successfully, he wishes that science would hurry up and solve his problems. Above all, he knows he needs help. He simply cannot keep abreast of the rapidly advancing frontier of medical knowledge.

The rapid increase in medical knowledge forces us to focus on two facts. The first is the lag between scientific discovery and its application in medical care. Serious attention has been given to this problem by our government, and legislation has been enacted to eliminate the lag in the treatment of patients suffering from heart disease, cancer, and stroke. The other fact is that a great deal of research and planning and many changes in our medical care system will have to take place if such legislation is to be effective. In order that the benefits of modern scientific knowledge be made available to all of our citizens, our plan for the future will take these two considerations seriously into account.

The dangerous complexities of modern medical care trouble dedicated physicians. The tools that are now in their hands are double edged. The old story attributed to Professor Lawrence J. Henderson in 1910 that "if the average patient visited the average physician, he would have a fifty-fifty chance of benefiting by the encounter" is no longer true. There was little specific treatment that a doctor could give his patient in 1910, and now he can do a great deal. But the tools of his trade — the potentially toxic drugs and the dramatic surgical techniques — can be both helpful and harmful. An adverse drug reaction may be more devastating than the underlying illness. An unwise decision as to surgical risk in a new and complex operation may cost the patient's life. There are also the accessory questions as to the optimum time to perform the surgery, how large a dose of drugs to administer, when to stop treatment, or when to increase the dose. It is a serious problem to balance the benefits and side effects of a complicated treatment with the natural history of a serious illness and to arrive at a precise decision as to what must be done for the patient. A careless, a poorly informed, or an exhausted physician could conceivably do more harm than good. But the wise, thoughtful, and informed physician can bring the miracles of modern medicine safely to his patients.

The Trend Toward Specialization

The more complicated things become, the more we need physicians to work in ever-narrowing areas; and as they concentrate their efforts, they become specialists. Moreover, as the explosion of biomedical knowledge is bound to continue, so will specialization become narrower and narrower, no matter what we try to do about it. Physicians must spend more time working in depth to give their patients the full advantage of medical knowledge and skills in the prevention and treatment of disease. Actually, the number of full-time specialists in the United States has increased about two and a half times during the last three decades, and the trend continues. We are fortunate that there has been such a remarkable evolution of specialization and an increase in the number and type of specialists in the United States. But there are not enough of all of them, and it is not likely that there ever will be enough to meet the needs of our unplanned society.

Specialists are scarce, and the growing demand for highly qualified specialists is not limited to medicine. It is symptomatic of the increasing complexity of our entire society. There is a real danger that our whole social structure will collapse because its complexities will outrun the supply of those needed to hold it together. In every field, professional, administrative, business, and government, there is an increasing deficit in the number of those needed to fill high-level positions. It is said that we do not have enough doctors, but it is apparent that there are also not enough physicists, engineers, nurses, or highly qualified technicians. I am sure we also agree that there are not enough competent people running for public office. But the situation is understandable. In our population, there is but a limited number of individuals with the combination of intelligence, originality, judgment, motivation, and wisdom necessary to leadership.

Specialization with its inherent rigidity has accentuated the deficit. The flexible adaptability of the natural philosopher has been lost. Benjamin Franklin, looking over his gold-rimmed spectacles, would have a frustrating time today attempting to learn enough in many fields to conduct his exciting and important experiments. In turn, specialization introduces rigidity and inflexibility into the entire system. Even in a grave emergency, an atomic scientist cannot take the place of a neurosurgeon at the operating table. Every field must be manned with both leaders and replacements.

Technology has also increased the demand for high-level personnel. If an automated machine is introduced to do laboratory tests, there will no longer be a need for technicians to suck on pipettes. But there will then be a search for more highly qualified technicians to supervise the machines. The intensive-care unit in the hospital decreases the need for ordinary nursing services but at the same time requires the most exacting competence in the nurse who will supervise the complicated equipment as well as the seriously ill patient. This trend cannot be continued indefinitely because there simply will not be enough people to provide the needed medical care. We shall be forced to analyze all of the tasks now performed by highly qualified personnel and identify those which truly demand their competence. In the same way, tasks conducted by such highly qualified personnel that do not call for a high degree of competence must be re-assigned to individuals with lesser but sufficient qualifications for these tasks.

The trend toward specialization has left another serious problem in its wake. Many of us have lost our personal physicians. Indeed, their numbers have decreased at about the same rate that the specialists have increased. We are faced with the question of where we are going to find a physician who will accept primary responsibility to provide continuity in our care and to give us personal health services and reassurance. It is a cruel illusion to believe that if we merely continue to build more and more medical schools or expand existing ones, and educate more and more medical students, we shall have more doctors of all of the kinds that are needed to take care of sick people. In fact, the recent increase in the number of medical graduates in the United States has supplied us with more specialists as the number of general physicians continues to decrease.

Spiraling Costs

The pressure of the spiraling costs of medical care is well known to all of us. As time goes on, it will be rare to find a family that has not had intimate experience with a medical problem that has threatened the structure of the family finances. Such personal experiences are reflected in the evidence provided by the Consumer Price Index. Between 1939 and 1960, the cost of medical care increased more than that of any other service, and of all items of care, hospital costs rose most sharply. These increased costs are already responsible for the growing demand for more complete medical care insurance coverage, particularly among those most vulnerable to disease — the very young and the very old — and among those whose incomes do not allow for the unpredictable and sometimes very large costs of severe illness.

The threat of hospital admission to a member of his family often causes great anxiety and strikes terror into the heart of the breadwinner. Hospital care is very costly. The explosion of knowledge and ever-narrowing specialization are represented in technical and medical advances that are expensive to supply. Hospital machinery is fantastically expensive, because the number of units sold will always remain relatively small. Moreover, space has to be found for the machines and they have to be operated and maintained by personnel of high competence.

Labor costs make up the largest item — more than two thirds — in the hospital budget, usually exceeding 70 per cent. There was a time when hospital employees, in the tradition of the charity care of the sick, were expected to contribute to the care of the patient by accepting lower wages than they would receive for equivalent work on the outside. But those days are long gone. Unionization has come to the hospital as it has to all industries, and the hospital must compete for its labor force.

The hospital does not have the flexibility of the industrial plant. The latter will add a night shift only if it proves profitable. But the hospital has no choice. It must operate twenty-four hours a day and meet increased demands at any hour of the day or night. Certain hospital personnel, particularly physicians, nurses, technicians, and maintenance workers have to be employed or be on call around the clock. As the industrial work week continues to shorten, the industrial plant can survive so long as increasing productivity compensates for it. It is clear that as long as medical advance progresses and the impact of labor costs continues to mount, hospital expenditures will continue to rise at an alarming rate.

Total health costs are reflected in the gross national product of our country. During the decade from 1955 to 1965, the proportion of gross national product spent on health services of all kinds shot up from 4.7 to about 6.1 per cent at a time when the gross national product itself was expanding at an unprecedented rate. It is reasonable to ask whether such a rate of growth in health costs can continue indefinitely.

In our affluent society we take for granted that every citizen is entitled to the benefits of any scientific fact, professional skill, and institutional resource that could promote health, prevent or treat disease or disability, or prevent untimely death. I would hope that in the future this will truly continue to be the case. Even though the increasing share of our gross national product that is allocated to health and medical care continues to increase, it is comparable with the mounting expenditures for space exploration or national defense. One could argue about the relative merits of expenditures for these purposes. Nevertheless, there is evidence that the cost of medical care cannot be expanded indefinitely. There must be a ceiling somewhere.

If we must embark upon the establishment of priorities and decide that we cannot bring all of medical science to all of our citizens, we immediately face many medical, practical, and ethical questions. A current example is the treatment of patients with an artificial organ. It is estimated that every year there are five thousand new cases of kidney failure that require treatment with the artificial kidney. At a cost of thousands of dollars for each patient and an undefined but lengthy period of years of treatment, it has been estimated that hundreds of millions of dollars will be needed annually to provide this one service. When the artificial heart becomes feasible, the cost can be expected to be even higher.

But cost cannot be the sole determining factor in establishing priorities. Potential medical benefits must be balanced against cost. Medical benefit comprises prevention, effective treatment, control of symptoms, and rehabilitation. Objective standards must be established by physicians and medical scientists in order to obtain reliable estimates of benefit to be balanced against the cost factors. In other words, even if cost factors finally force us to set up priorities of medical care with the understanding that those at the bottom of the list will not be funded, we must have the scientific knowledge necessary for sound decisions.

One word of caution. Medical benefits cannot be based on the undocumented statements of prominent physicians nor on the effectiveness of their political lobbying. The first step is to find out what really can be done. It is not enough, for example, for the President's Commission on Heart Disease, Cancer, and Stroke to look at mortality figures and say that these are the three major causes of death. Such figures cannot be used to discriminate between those patients in whom such an illness is merely a terminal event — or cannot be treated — and those in whom it is a cause of preventable death — or can be treated.

Social benefits must also be taken into account. Our current emphasis on artificial organs and national programs to aid those suffering from heart disease, cancer, and stroke is focused on chronic illnesses and on patients in the middle and older age groups. Such an emphasis is in sharp contrast with that in England during World War II, where the major question was survival. The health of children and pregnant women was given highest priority. The children were sent out of London, given most of the available nutritious foods such as eggs and milk, and fed jam made of rose hips — the only available source of Vitamin C. Pregnant women were given special consideration and rations of scarce nutritious foods. In our country, if funds available for medical care become limited, should they be spent mostly on decreasing our infant mortality with its estimated annual excess of 40,000 deaths[7] or should they be concentrated on prolonging the lives of the aged?

[7] William H. Stewart, Surgeon General of the United States

Such questions are not farfetched. They have already been posed. A few years ago *The Wall Street Journal*[8] reported that the State of Colorado, having exhausted its $10 million appropriation for old-age medical care before the end of the fiscal year, suspended payments until the next year's budget became available and "barred oldsters from entering hospitals except in emergencies." Surely a decision as to the cessation of hospital care should not depend on the exhaustion of the budget. If funds are limited, such decisions should be predicated on a priority list of relative benefits of medical procedures, based on medical knowledge interpreted by medical scientists and physicians.

The pressure of spiraling costs is not an unmitigated evil. It will force us to re-examine the structure of medical practice and evaluate the relative effectiveness of medical procedures. It is here that leadership must be provided by the medical profession. Both politics and statesmanship are involved: politics because government is so deeply concerned, statesmanship because wise direction is necessary. Indeed, accepting the definition of politics as the art of the possible and defining statesmanship as the science of the necessary, the medical profes-

---

Public Health Service, gave this estimate at the meeting of the American Academy of Pediatrics, Chicago, Ill., October 24, 1966, on the basis that the United States rate could be as low as the infant mortality rate of Sweden.

[8] James Harwood, "Health Plan's Ills, "*The Wall Street Journal*, June 9, 1961.

sion must identify the necessary and convince the public, and through them the politicians, that it is possible. Unfortunately, at the present time the medical profession is exerting very little leadership. As a consequence of the bloody battle over Medicare legislation and the negative position assumed by organized medicine, there is a lack of adequate representation for medicine in Washington and in the state capitals. Until there is, the public through their political representatives will be forced to make medical care decisions without adequate guidance.

Changing Public Expectations

The pressure of rising public expectations has had a significant effect on medical care. The public's concept of medicine and disease has changed. Disease is no longer thought to be punishment for sin. Now, you "can do something about it." People once went to the hospital when they were too sick to be cared for at home. Or, they would not go because it was "the place you went to die." With the impact of science on daily life and the development of "miracle drugs" and dramatic operations, people now go to the hospital to receive the benefits of the technology of medicine.

The great expansion in the science and technology of medicine has been reflected in public attitudes. On television, for example, we no longer see the old doctor with a gray beard walking through the snow in the middle of the night carrying a black bag on his way to deliver a baby. Instead, we see a young physician, always in the hospital, surrounded by pretty nurses, carrying out a highly complicated technical procedure during which the patient's life hangs by a thread. The background for the physician is a hospital scene furnished in glass, chromium, and stainless steel and decorated with festoons of plastic tubing and the flashing lights of electronic equipment.

The specialist and his technology keynote modern medical care. Moreover, the specialist working with his hands is more appreciated than the thoughtful physician curing his patient without the help of mechanical aids. The public is more impressed by manual dexterity than by a brilliant diagnosis, and this is understandable. Action is almost always more impressive than words. This attitude is reflected in the way the public pays for its medical services. The parent understands that the open-heart surgical operation on his child may require a mortgage on his home. But if the fee he pays to his general doctor is increased by $5.00 for one visit, he will complain and grumble.

Abetted by sensational articles in the popular press and in the annual fund-raising drives of national health agencies and by the promises from medical spokesmen of the imminent solution to our major medical problems, the public has begun to expect far too much from his doctor, from the hospital, and from medicine. The public has been oversold. Even the most staid and accurate newspapers carry front-page reports on break-throughs in the control of major illnesses at regular intervals. Thus, responsible publications cure cancer almost every week. At fund-raising time, spokesmen for our great national health agencies clearly imply that all that is lacking is money and that if enough were made available the "big answer" would be just around the corner. Scientists, being human, tend to be overly optimistic about the implications of their research results. All of this creates extravagant public expectations and often cruelly raises and dashes the hopes of sufferers from mortal illnesses.

The public is also misled about its own medical care. Patients are often not satisfied with less than their version of the latest treatment. Physicians now spend a great deal of time reassuring patients as they destroy false hopes engendered by careless public statements. This public attitude has and will continue to place great pressure on the individual physician and the hospital to do the impossible, that is, to try to provide the public's concept of medical care.

This public attitude also seriously affects the research scientist. He is constantly interrupted and tempted by demands for an immediate public announcement of his recent discovery as he labors patiently collecting his research data — without which great medical advances are practically impossible.

Overselling of the public has also been reflected in the

medical care budget. Needless visits to the doctor and time spent in reassurance of the patient disturbed by carelessly worded news releases are wasteful of both the physician's time and the public's money. Moreover, the purchase of an unnecessary but dramatic piece of complicated equipment, such as a cobalt bomb in the local community hospital under pressure from a trustee or a prominent patient, builds up the deficit in the hospital budget.

Public interest, knowledge, and support are all necessary to the progress of medicine. With carefully designed public education programs under professional leadership, the current unreasonable public expectations and confused demands could be guided into productive channels.

Depersonalization

During the past few decades, the progressive depersonalization of our society has placed great stress on our haphazard system of medical care. To be sure, depersonalization in medicine is but one manifestation of the great depersonalization of our entire society. Depersonalization has resulted from the interaction of the many social changes, which has led to progressive urbanization with many more very young and very old people crowded into our cities. In the name of efficiency we are forced into progressive expanding industrialization with lockstep assembly lines, factories in the field, unwieldy labor unions, and faceless corporations.

In the suburbs of our small towns with their stereotyped main streets, choked with traffic and lined with chain stores, there is a supermarket where the corner grocery once stood but no butcher, tailor, or shoemaker shop. The assembly line monotony is manifested externally by the boring sameness of female dress in every hamlet and metropolis from coast to coast. Our burgeoning overpopulation has accelerated depersonalization, because survival under crowded conditions demands repetitive systematic organization to a point where personal services become relatively ineffective and it becomes "cheaper to throw it away and buy a new one."

The lack of personal service frustrates us when we cannot find a reliable, interested repairman for our television set or obtain personal attention from the meat-counter clerk so busy stamping purple prices on plastic-wrapped frankfurters. For better or for worse, we tolerate in the name of efficiency all of these manifestations of depersonalization, including the loss of many personal health services.

But we cannot permit this trend, as efficient as it may become, to further depersonalize medical care. The price is too great. The words "medical care" imply personal attention and service, the loss of which may be more than frustrating. It may cost the life or health of the patient, as sometimes occurs when physicians are not available at nights or on weekends.

Progressive depersonalization in medical care will certainly result in the deterioration of the physician-patient relationship. Specialization itself creates depersonalization. As we continue to specialize, and if no one physician assumes total responsibility for the patient, we shall have an increasing loss of continuity in patient care. We must be more efficient and yet maintain the personal relationship between physician and patient. We must not sacrifice tender loving care.

Impact and Resolution of the Paradox

The paradox of modern medicine has produced both personal and scientific disquietude. There is unhappiness on every side about the way in which medical care is provided.

The patient has many complaints: the delays in relief of pain and suffering because physicians are often unavailable, the anxieties incurred by weeks of waiting for an appointment with a physician or for a hospital bed, and the near impossibility of finding a nurse to bring comfort during convalescence. Worst of all, our slum dwellers put up with interminable waits in poorly furnished, inadequately equipped clinics, with a loss of the day's pay for a brief and unsatisfactory visit with the physician, and with the unnecessary burden and anguish of preventable illness and of too many dying babies.

Our doctors are overworked. They properly complain of unnecessary demands upon their time and are overwhelmed by the increasing complexity of their tasks as they attempt to bring the benefits of modern medical care to their patients. They are also anxious about the specter of social change that could deprive them of their economic status as entrepreneurs.

Hospitals are crowded and are struggling to balance their budgets. Many hospital units remain closed or operate dangerously because of the inability to maintain an adequate nursing staff. The enactment of Medicare legislation that has almost eliminated the economic barrier to acute hospital care for our older citizens has accentuated the crisis. Waiting lists for admission to our general hospitals are becoming progressively longer. The almost complete lack of modern medical facilities for the care of the chronically ill outside the acute general hospital makes it more and more difficult to discharge patients no longer needing intensive treatment but whose very lives may depend upon good follow-up care.

Nurses are dissatisfied with their present tasks and are confused by the variety of demands that are being made upon them. At one moment the "nurse" may be expected to carry serious professional responsibilities in monitoring the reaction of a patient to a powerful drug or in supervising the facilities in the operating room for a life-saving surgical procedure. At the very next moment the "nurse" may be expected to perform the menial task of cleaning up the bed of the patient incontinent of urine and feces.

Medical schools are having great difficulty in defining their objectives. The deans and their faculties are squeezed between the increasing rigorousness of complex science and technology in their research programs and the demands of society for an increase in the number of practicing physicians who will have as their major interest the welfare of their patients.

The paradox of modern medicine must be resolved. Scientific advance must continue without interruption and yet must be matched with concomitant improvement in medical care. The pressures that have brought us to this state of affairs are many and powerful. Little can be done about most of them but all can be harnessed and directed toward the evolution of a better program for medical care in the future.

The Tangled Web of Medical Care

The web of medical care is both tangled and torn. The catch-as-catch-can structure of our unplanned medical care system is comprised of conflicting and duplicating activities on the one hand and gaps in service on the other. Doctors settle where they will with large numbers in the suburbs and few, if any, in the country or in the slums of our large cities. Hospital centers tend to be self-centered. Their growth in buildings and equipment is usually determined not by community need but by financial resources, the interest and demands of the medical staff, and the pride and drive of the board of trustees. Public health and social service resources appear to grow with the social outlook of the community, with more and better services in the wealthier communities and fewer and poorer services in the low-income areas where they are most needed. All of these discrepancies persist even though our federal government through legislation and financial allocations attempts to equalize services throughout the country.

The hallmark of our present haphazard system of medical care is lack of efficient systematic allocation of resources to meet the public need. Implicit is a lack of planning, which really reflects the pitiful inadequacy of research on the provision of medical care. Indeed, our blind faith in the infallibility of the physician has made it seem in the past as if research on medical care were unnecessary. But now, unhappily, the tangled state in which we find our medical care demands that we do something about it. If our planning is to be effective, we must examine and evaluate the methods by which medical care is provided as precisely as we investigate the mechanisms of the diseases we wish to prevent and treat.

Operations Research

Fortunately, a body of knowledge and techniques known as "operations research" is being developed that is directly applicable to the study of medical care. In essence, operations research is useful in any situation where there are limited resources available to satisfy a complex need. Historically, operations research was first used in the deployment of troops and matériel in World War II. The success of operations research in military logistics led to the extension of its use to industrial production problems in war industry, then to industrial problems in general, to business management, and to economic planning. Now it is being applied to public health and medical care. In a policy statement on operations research prepared for the World Health Organization with Professors Marcel-Paul Schutzenberger and Murray Eden, we pointed out that operations research is useful in the kinds of major decisions that frequently face the medical administrator. They are as follows:

1. How does one assess the relative needs for, and the values of, alternative programs that must draw upon limited resources in funds, matériel, and trained manpower?

2. How shall available resources be best allocated and applied once a decision on priorities has been made?

These same questions have been successfully answered in military situations and in industry. In public health a beginning has been made, for instance in the tuberculosis control program of the World Health Organization for India. Operations research analysis of many possible applications of the limited health resources and manpower supported an immunization program for babies with BCG vaccine rather than the search for and isolation of the infectious cases.

It is essential for the solution of many of our major medical care problems that existing operations research knowledge and techniques be effectively used. Moreover, new theory will have to be developed to satisfy the special requirements of medical care as well as of biomedical problems. For example, the application of inventory theory to blood banks will require that the perishable nature of human red-blood cells be taken into account. In documenting the uses of operations research in medical care, and as a background for the "Plan for the Medicine of the Future," we shall first examine the medical manpower problem and then the nature of the social and administrative structure in which medical care is provided.

Medical Manpower

As we look into the future, we see that the physician is changing from an individual practitioner working alone to the central figure in a constellation consisting of many different kinds of other medical and nonmedical workers. Whatever his change in role, I cannot visualize a satisfactory system of medical care in which a physician will not have a close personal relationship with his patient. For his part, the patient must be able to place his trust in his doctor. Moreover, some one individual must direct and be responsible for the complex personal service called medical care. The confused, perplexed patient must know to whom he can turn for guidance and support. I realize that many other solutions have been proposed, but as I look at the issue from the patient's point of view I see no substitute for the physician as the focal point in the constellation of medical care.

Let us accept the fact that a physician can no longer practice alone. Both the general physician and specialist now know that they must have expensive, complicated equipment and facilities if medical care is to include the benefits of recent advances in science and technology. As a result, physicians are joined together in ever more comprehensive group practice units,[1] which in turn are developing a closer and closer relationship to the locus of medical technology — the modern hospital.

But physicians, even when grouped together in the most efficient ways with the best of hospital and other medical facilities accessible to them, cannot by themselves provide us with up-to-date medical care. Many others must help them. Indeed, there are many different kinds of people in the medical constellation who assist the doctor, ranging all the way from professional personnel to manual laborers.

The Other Health Professions

First we have the health professions — the college-educated, professionally trained, group of health workers. A member of a health profession has accepted responsibility for an area of activity, has followed a special course of study usually leading to a degree, and has met the established requirements for licensure. Included in this category are nurses, medical social workers, dietitians, nurse-midwives, pharmacists, hospital and public health administrators, laboratory, X-ray, and many other

[1] The term group practice is used to mean the cooperative organization of physicians to conduct a particular medical care plan as, for example, the Kaiser Permanente Plan in California or the Health Insurance Plan of Greater New York. Group practice is not the mere sharing of facilities for economic reasons alone, for example, dividing the cost of an examining room or of a laboratory or paying jointly for the services of a secretary.

kinds of technicians, and physical, speech, occupational, hearing, and other kinds of therapists. Members of the health professions have implicitly accepted a degree of individual responsibility that may directly affect the life or health of the patient.

New categories of health professions are frequently being created, such as those of supertechnicians for servicing artificial organs, nurse monitors for intensive care units, and systems analysts to bring modern management into medical care. The health professions have expanded in number, in membership, and in scope in a completely haphazard way, and duplications and gaps in services to the patient have been the result. The number of health professional workers has increased at an astounding rate from about 75 thousand in 1900 to an estimated 900 thousand in 1960.

The Health Vocations

Now we turn to the three quarters of a million health vocational workers. Health vocational workers provide nontechnical services to or conduct supervised procedures practically always for the patient, as for example, the preparation of a patient prior to a surgical operation. The vocational group includes such workers as practical nurses, nurses' aides, orderlies, attendants, and laboratory assistants. The health vocational worker performs tasks demanding special skills. He is trained to perform such tasks competently under general supervision.

Members of the health professions and vocations are usually referred to as *ancillary medical personnel,* since they are closely related to the physician to whom they are ultimately responsible.

Nonmedical Employees in the Health Industry

Another category, not included under ancillary medical personnel, comprises nonmedical workers employed in the health industry. Examples are drug manufacturing employees, pharmacists' clerks, ambulance drivers, the electricians, plumbers, other maintenance workers, the housekeeping staff members in the hospital, and the secretaries of physicians. For obvious reasons, the boundaries of this group are difficult to define. It has been conservatively estimated that there are at least two million nonmedical workers employed in the health industry.

Collaborative Professions

In addition to the constellation of personnel surrounding and responsible to the physician are the professions that collaborate directly with him in research, education, and medical care. Some examples are bioscientists, biochemists, X-ray crystallographers, medical economists, and demographers. We are at the moment concerned with the engineer as he collaborates with the physician in bringing new basic sciences, operations research, automation, and technology into medicine and biology.

This evolving relationship depends on each profession recognizing and respecting the contribution of the other and on their collaboration as equals.

In developing a relationship between the physician and members of other professions, we can learn much from the failures of the past. The failure of physicians and architects to work together in the design of a hospital is the classical case. One might reasonably expect that the first step in the design of a hospital would be a precise statement of the program of activities to be conducted within its walls. But such has not usually been the case. Medical guidance has often been limited to the names of the services to be housed, for example, pediatrics, or the number of operating rooms in surgery rather than to the precise tasks to be performed and the flow of activity to be expected. Such failure has usually forced the architect to design a hospital that satisfies his ideas of medical care rather than those of the physician. For his part, the architect, seeing little possibility of close collaboration with the physician in the design of a hospital, fails to call attention to newer architectural materials or designs that might relieve the physician from structural limitations that have plagued him in the past. The results of this lack of collaboration are documented by glaring deficiencies in the already outmoded structures of newly built hospitals throughout the country. An interesting exception is the International Center for Technical Studies in Paris that has pioneered in the solution of this problem by making every effort to bring together the medical and architectural professions in the planning for and the designing of a hospital.

Whatever the profession working together with medicine, true collaboration requires that each profession analyze the problem from its point of view and then join with the other in an exchange of ideas and information, and then repeat the process as each step is completed along the way. Depending upon the problem at hand, the initiative at one moment may rest with the physician while at the next it may rest with, for example, the demographer, the engineer, the economist, or the biochemist.

The Image Is a Lone Physician

It is almost painfully obvious that a large number of all kinds of personnel are needed to help the doctor. But when we plan for the future, we only too often act as if he provides medical care all by himself. We plan, finance, and build more and bigger medical schools, we design new medical curricula and hope to graduate more doctors, and give little or no consideration to the changing role of the physician — from that of a lone practitioner to that of the central figure in a wide and heavily populated constellation of professional and vocational medical workers. Indeed, in the recently published "Millis

Report"[2] there is but one brief reference to ancillary medical personnel. The fiction carries on.

As a result of this naïve attitude, we use the number of doctors available to a particular population as a major index of the adequacy of medical care, with the physician/population ratio as the standard measurement. There must, of course, be a maximum number of people to be cared for by a single physician no matter how efficient the system of medical care. A physician/population ratio of from 1:7,000 up to 1:190,000 in the countries on the continent of Africa (except Egypt and the Union of South Africa) is obviously too small.[3] But in the United States, where the national rate is about one physician for every 750 people, the range of variation among the fifty states extends from 1:280 to 1:1,400 people and the ratios, as we shall see, are almost meaningless.

The physician/population ratio does not take into account many important characteristics of modern medical progress. It tells us the total number of physicians in a particular population, with the implicit assumption that all of them are in full-time private practice. It thus does not allow for the increasing proportion of licensed physicians who are concentrating full time in other endeav-

[2] *The Graduate Education of Physicians*, a Citizen's Committee Report, sponsored by the American Medical Association, 1966.

[3] *Union Africaine et Malgache de Coopération Economique.* Etude monographique de 31 pays africains, Vol. 1 (1964), Paris.

ors. For example, I am a specialist in internal medicine, but because I work full time in a medical school I see very few patients other than those on the services of the teaching hospitals. And yet I am counted in the ratio in the same way as the physician who spends all of his professional time giving individual patient care.

The ratio treats specialists and general physicians as if they provided similar services. Moreover, it does not distinguish among the specialties nor assure an appropriate balance among them. In some communities there might be, for example, a complete absence of certain specialists such as neurosurgeons or too many of others such as general surgeons.

The physician/population ratio in any geographic area does not allow for their concentration in the suburbs and their scarcity in rural areas and in the poorer sections of our larger cities. The ratio assumes that all physicians are equally accessible to all people in the area and does not take geographic and economic barriers into account.

Quality is also neglected. All physicians, regardless of their education, training, experience, and competence, are treated alike in the calculation of the ratio.

Finally, since the ratio assumes that the physician acts alone, it disregards the efficiency of the system in which he practices his profession. Indeed, the ratio implies that the physician's services are completely independent of hospital and other facilities and that he needs no help from other medical personnel. It makes no allowance for the concept that the physician is the focal point in an intricate constellation of medical institutions, resources, and personnel.

There are curious inconsistencies when actual physician/population ratios are compared with the local health status in particular areas. Allowing for the leveling off of our health indices, it is still true that the greatest advances in the history of medicine have taken place in the last half century. And yet, the physician/population ratio in the United States has remained relatively constant at a level of about 1 doctor to 750 persons. It is obvious that the index gives us little inkling of improvement in medical care. Indeed, in the first decade of this century when medical education was haphazard and uncontrolled and medical care was consequently very poor, there was a higher ratio of doctors (1 for every 560 people) than there is now.

There are other incongruities. In 1950, South Dakota had the lowest ratio of physicians to population (1 to 1,400) among the forty-eight states. And yet, in that state, in the same year, white males had a longer life expectancy than they had in any other state (68.4 years).

In direct contrast, in 1964, the District of Columbia had the highest ratio of nonfederal physicians[4] to popu-

---

[4] Federal physicians, that is, members of the Armed Forces, the Veteran's Administration, and the United States Public Health Service, including the National Institutes of Health, are excluded from this ratio.

lation (about 1 to 280). But the District of Columbia in the same year had the highest neonatal mortality rate (deaths of newborns during the first four weeks of life) of any of the fifty states. The District of Columbia was also in that same year second only to Mississippi in the height of its infant mortality rate (deaths of newborns during the first year of life) in the United States.

It is clear that a "favorable" physician/population ratio does not necessarily correlate with the highest standards of health. Of course, there must be a critical number of physicians below which medical care cannot be provided. But the facts indicate that at the level of the present physician/population ratio in the United States other factors are probably more important to the welfare of the patient than the ratio of doctors to population in a given geographic area. In the United States the physician/population ratio is therefore not a valid index of the adequacy of medical care.

Since it is clear that the physician does not act alone, we must examine his role in our complex system of medical care in order to plan for the future. If his role can be precisely defined, we should be able to help him provide better medical care in three different ways. An analysis of his tasks will permit the delegation to others of those that do not demand his background, education, knowledge, skills, and experience. Operations research can help by designing a more effective system in which he can care for his patients. Third, automation and technology can increase his productivity and perhaps aid him in bringing medical care to his patients.

Specialists and General Practitioners

There are two major groups of physicians — those called "general practitioners" and specialists. With the explosion of knowledge and the consequent increase in the number of specialists, the number of general practitioners has been decreasing. Actually, physicians calling themselves general practitioners decreased in numbers in the United States from about 112,000 in 1931 to 82,000 in 1959. The trend continues. In a study in 1961 by the Department of Preventive Medicine at the Harvard Medical School, under the direction of Dr. Osler L. Peterson,[5] of the graduates of medical school classes of 1950 and 1954 in twelve representative medical schools, the downward trend could be discerned even for that short interval. Indeed, it continues through December 1966.[6] Fewer medical graduates are now going into general practice.

[5] Osler L. Peterson, Fremont J. Lyden, H. Jack Geiger, and Theodore Colton, "Appraisal of Medical Students' Abilities as Related to Training and Careers After Graduation," *The New England Journal of Medicine*, 269 (November 28, 1963), 1174–1182.

[6] Ivan Fahs and Osler Peterson, "Medical Care and the Decline of General Practice," An Addendum to the Millis Report (in process of publication).

The trends that led inevitably to specialization are understandable. The research worker, using increasingly complex techniques, penetrated deeper into ever-narrowing fields of investigation. In turn, the practicing physician who wanted to take advantage of the expanding reservoir of knowledge was forced to add years to his training and to limit his scope to specific organ systems — such as the nervous system — or to patterns of illness — such as, for instance, allergic diseases. The emergence of specialists was encouraged by the patients' immediate acceptance of the expert and their willingness to pay more for his services than for those of a general physician.

The expert knowledge and skills of the specialist were sorely needed. They provided the basis for the growing reputation of American medicine. But, as early as 1927, thoughtful physicians such as Francis Peabody recognized that the very process of specialization created new and serious gaps. By its nature, the specialist's care was confined to a particular part or special illness of the patient. Indeed, the same symptoms might fall within the purview of more than one specialist. For instance, a severe pain in your left shoulder for which you (mistakenly) consult an orthopedic surgeon might be due to heart disease, which would require treatment by a cardiologist. Absorbed with the mechanism of disease, the specialist sometimes neglects to relieve the very symptoms that brought you to his office. Drugs to ease the back pain may be forgotten as both surgeon and radiologist concentrate on that clear shadow in your X-ray films.

Moreover, by focusing on his particular field of interest, one specialist might miss a manifestation of serious illness within the preserve of another. The cardiac consultant, listening to the sounds coming through a stethoscope, might very well overlook that small lump in your breast that you accidentally discover four months later after it has grown a bit larger.

As specialties have multiplied and narrowed, several doctors may be caring for the same patient and yet not cover all of his health problems. If a single physician does not accept responsibility for all aspects of the patient's care, the opposite situation may also occur; the treatment prescribed by one specialist may conflict with that of another. Indeed, coordination of services and continuity of treatment have become strikingly deficient even in some of our great teaching hospitals.

In the meantime, what has happened to the family doctor? His prestige, particularly in urban areas of the United States, has been gradually downgraded. Examining boards created to certify specialists have established a hierarchy of practitioners above him. As the care of serious disease has shifted from the home to the hospital, hospital services have been gradually reshaped to conform with the trends in specialization. Better highways and more automobiles have made transportation to office and to hospital relatively easy, so that home visits except in an emergency have become increasingly rare. The family physician not qualified in a specialty has an increasingly difficult time obtaining a hospital appointment. This has lowered his status in the eyes of the patient, who on admission to the hospital will be cared for by another physician — the specialist.

Thus the general physician has lost status in the eyes of both his profession and the public. To be sure, we cannot and do not wish to resurrect the "old family doctor" practicing all alone, isolated from specialists and from the hospital and working without the assistance of paramedical personnel and without modern technical equipment. Nevertheless, we must face the fact that medical care in the United States is suffering from the lack of general physicians or other mechanisms to accept primary responsibility for the patient, to provide continuity in his care, and to give him personal health services and reassurance.

In 1960, I suggested one possible solution to this difficult problem.[7] To allow for the admission and education of general physicians, present admission policies that favor the selection of students suitable for careers of research scientists and specialists must, of course, be continued and strengthened. But, in addition, new admission criteria must be established for acceptance of

[7] A proposal for an additional medical curriculum to educate the general physician. David D. Rutstein, "Do You Really Want a Family Doctor?" *Harper's Magazine*, Oct. 1960, pp. 144–150.

students looking toward a career as general physicians. Medical schools would recognize that the education of the family physician in modern dress demands a curriculum that must be scientifically based but must also be designed to meet the needs of a general physician rather than those of the more esoteric, more narrowly focused specialist career now embraced by the large majority of medical graduates.

When this same proposal was presented to the Association of American Medical Colleges[8] it was greeted by a howl of pain from the deans of American medical schools, who promptly reassured each other that there really was no problem because internists and pediatricians would meet the needs. Obviously, when they are available, internists and pediatricians tend to do a superb job of providing general medical care, but there is only one internist for about every 14,000 people in the United States, they are crowded in the suburbs of our more affluent cities, and one third of all of them practice in the two states of New York and California.

The deans were warned by outstanding leaders of American medical education that the major effect of such a plan would be to lower the standards of American

[8] David D. Rutstein, "Physicians For Americans—Two Medical Curricula," *Journal of Medical Education*, Vol. 36 Supplement, *Medical Education and Medical Care, Interactions and Prospects* (December 1961), pp. 129–138.

medicine.[9] To be sure, a proposal for two separate medical curricula in each medical school sounded naïve at a time when a single, rigid medical curriculum was the only way to educate a medical student. Of course, this occurred before the currently recognized need for a more flexible medical curriculum to meet the widening spectrum of career opportunities for graduates of medical schools. Indeed, as we shall see, we now recognize that we must tailor the medical curriculum to meet the needs of every medical student, including those who wish to become general physicians.

What has happened in the interval since 1960? Needless to say, nothing was done and we have been forced to improvise. Most of the physicians now going into general practice in the United States, indeed, one out of every five physicians now being licensed for the first time in one of our states, is a graduate of a foreign medical school, most often in developing countries such as the Philippines, Iran, India, Turkey, and Mexico. These are all countries that can ill afford to supply physicians to us. Indeed, we ought to be producing a surplus of doctors, beyond our own needs, to send to underdeveloped areas — as the Russians are already doing.

[9] Dana W. Atchley, "The Vanishing Family Doctor," Letter to the Editor, *Harper's Magazine*, December 1960, pp. 80–81; William Barry Wood, *From Miasmas To Molecules*, Bampton Lectures No. 13 (New York: Columbia University Press, 1961).

By default others have taken over the duties of the general physician. The approximately fifteen thousand osteopaths are taking the place of the disappearing general physician. In urban areas, patients throng the emergency rooms of the larger hospitals to obtain the services of a physician. Such care, given by a member of the rapidly changing intern and resident staff who may be on duty at the moment, can only be episodic and relatively impersonal. The general hospital has thus assumed a heavy load of ambulatory medical care.

To meet rural needs, states, including New York and Massachusetts, have enacted legislation to license chiropractors. Apparently, it is easier to get a bad law enacted by a state legislature than a new idea implemented by a medical faculty. In both urban and rural areas, the local druggist has become the medical adviser. We may have reasonable doubts whether all of these efforts have succeeded in maintaining high standards of medical care in the United States. But it is clear that the ivory towers of most of our academic medical institutions have been safely protected from the community need for general health services.

Reallocation of Medical Tasks

In our present system of medical practice, physicians, nurses, and members of other medical professional groups are in short supply. If some tasks could be delegated to others with fewer qualifications, more professional time would become available for those tasks that *do* demand the competence of the physician. All physicians' tasks will have to be examined individually to determine which do not demand his qualifications. In turn, the individual tasks of members of the other medical professions must be studied in the same way to determine which may be delegated to vocational medical personnel.

Let us examine how this process has already affected the role of the nurse. When I was a house officer at the Boston City Hospital in the 1930's, needle punctures could be performed only by a physician, with but one exception: a nurse could inject a prescribed drug under the skin. She was not permitted to insert a needle into a vein.

In the late 1940's, after nurses had been forced by the war emergency to take on previously forbidden tasks, some hospitals permitted them to draw blood from, but not to inject medication into, a vein. Now, in hospitals such as the Massachusetts General Hospital, a small group of specially trained nurses gives all intravenous treatment, including drugs, fluids, and transfusions, while technicians collect blood specimens for analysis. Most important, they perform these tasks much more efficiently and with more skill than was previously demonstrated by the average physician.

Allocation of increasing technical responsibility to nonphysicians will certainly continue. The nurse or a specially trained supertechnician will soon be collecting specimens of spinal fluid and tapping abnormal accumulations of chest or abdominal fluid. Eventually, she will be incising boils and draining simple abscesses. In effect, mechanical procedures of ever-increasing technical difficulty will be delegated by the physician to other medical personnel. In turn, many tasks performed by nurses will be delegated to vocational personnel.

Nursing now covers such a wide range and so overlaps the activities of other professions, such as that of the medical social workers, that it deserves special analysis and a redefinition of roles within the profession itself. This undertaking is made ever more difficult by confused terminology. The recent position paper of the American Nursing Association[10] refers to such titles as professional nurse, professional practitioner, technical nurse, nurse, nurse-practitioner, registered nurse, licensed practical nurse, nurses' aide, orderly, assistant, and attendant.

In order to untangle this portion of the web, let us examine the different kinds of competences now included within the generic term "nurse." We shall start with examples of those nursing tasks demanding the highest level of professional and administrative responsibility. Included would be directors of hospitals and public health nursing units and directors of nursing schools. Also, in certain rural areas, the public health nurse ac-

---

[10] "American Nurses' Association's First Position on Education for Nursing," *American Journal of Nursing*, 65 (December 1965), 106–111.

cepts responsibility very close to that of the general physician. Indeed, she often acts as his emissary. She interprets the physician's instructions within the practical limitations of the patient's environment, reinforces self-education of immediate applicability, administers prescribed injections or collects specimens for laboratory examinations, identifies new health and medical care problems, supplies personal attention and reassuring comfort to the patient, and relays information back to the patient's physician. In urban areas, the nurse in charge of an intensive care unit in a hospital literally holds the patients' lives in her hands as she monitors the control panel. All of these tasks require extensive educational background and acceptance of independent responsibility.

The next category includes those who have immediate and serious supervisory responsibilities. The nurse in charge of a hospital ward must identify sudden changes in the patient's condition due to his disease or to such other causes as an adverse drug reaction. In the operating room, the surgical nurse must provide the sterile facilities, equipment, and environment so that the surgeon may perform his operation with safety and ease. Nurses with supervisory responsibilities must, under general supervision, make immediate judgments that may affect the life or health of the patient. Their technical education must be adequate for such tasks and they must be trained to make rapid and precise decisions.

The average staff nurse performs the dual role of providing professional services, such as the administration of a drug, and the menial tasks involved in keeping a patient comfortable and clean. In smaller hospitals she may at times perform housekeeping tasks, although these are now carried out mostly by practical nurses or ward maids. The education of the staff nurse must include knowledge of important symptoms and signs of illness so that she may detect a patient in difficulty at the earliest possible moment.

All of these professional nursing groups are assisted by the large number of vocational workers who are concerned with the comfort and hygiene of the patient. Included are licensed practical nurses and nurses' aides.

The single word "nurse" appears in all of the titles included in this wide range of activity. As a result, there is confusion in status and everyone concerned with nursing is unhappy. The doctor complains that the nurse does too much paper work and not enough direct care. The hospital administrator complains that the records are incomplete. The patient complains that he cannot get a nurse "when he needs one." The poor nurse herself is bewildered, and her motivation to be an "angel of mercy" is undermined.

The confusion in status has resulted in salary scales appropriate to the less demanding nursing activities. Salaries now paid to "nurses" are almost at the level of bedpan carriers. According to a report of the United

States Bureau of Labor Statistics, in 1963–1964 class-room teachers averaged $6,235 a year, secretaries $5,170, and factory workers $5,075. In the same period, general duty nurses in nonfederal city hospitals, the largest group of nurses, averaged $4,500 per year.

The Structure of Medical Care

The structure in which medical personnel provide medical care is made up of many different kinds of inter-acting units, including hospitals, nursing homes, Blue Cross, Blue Shield, and private insurance companies, the Social Security Administration, the United States Public Health Service, the state and local health departments, and voluntary health and welfare agencies including those concerned with special diseases. I shall examine the hospital because it is a good example for our purposes. Its evolution epitomizes, in effect, the changes in the total structure of our medical care program.

During the first half of the twentieth century the hospital changed from a custodial institution to a complex workshop.[11] Now, the hospital has already become the focal point for medical care. This is fortunate. By examining the assets and liabilities for medical care within the hospital, we can see with our own eyes the essential

[11] David D. Rutstein, "At the Turn of the Next Century," Lowell Lecture delivered at the Massachusetts General Hospital on May 15, 1963.

characteristics of our entire medical care system. There are many examples: the haphazard state of medical care within the United States is illustrated by the lack of coordination among our many different kinds of hospitals and the detached, independent operation of the individual hospital. Such disorganization may, in fact, be a major weakness in the structure of our medical care system because we are a nation of small hospitals. We, in Boston, accustomed to large urban hospitals, are surprised to learn that more than 60 per cent of the hospitals in our country have fewer than one hundred beds, and more than a third have fewer than fifty beds. The wide distribution of small hospitals throughout the country is the heritage of the Hill-Burton Act that provided federal funds for hospitals, each of which was expected to be self-sufficient.

Because of the haphazard distribution and the relatively small size of most of our hospitals, it is simply impossible — indeed foolish — to equip and staff all of them to provide every specialized service. But this idea is not new. In the United States the concept is already established that every general hospital cannot provide every service to every patient. For example, complicated lifesaving equipment, such as the artificial kidney, needed only by an occasional patient, is available in relatively few hospitals. It has also been evident for a very long time that the laboratories of every hospital cannot perform all tests. Complicated, unusual, and dangerous laboratory tests are farmed out to laboratories in other hospitals or in state health departments or to unique laboratories such as that of the Communicable Disease Center of the United States Public Health Service in Atlanta, Georgia.

In epidemic emergencies, hospital resources have been centralized for their more effective use. During the polio epidemic in metropolitan Boston in 1955, three hospitals were selected to treat all the patients under the supervision of a few eminent specialists. The patients received superb care.

The wasteful duplication of specialist resources in our hospitals is documented by the almost endless proliferation of highly specialized services, for example, heart surgery in some of our large cities. This is in sharp contrast with the practice in Sweden, where superspecialists' services are created and located in accordance with the need. Thus, in 1953, there was but one radium treatment center — Radiumhemmet in the Karolinska Hospital in Stockholm. In 1963, by the time of my next visit, there were five centers distributed over the country and there was some discussion that a sixth might be needed. In 1966, there were six radium treatment centers in Sweden and some discussion of the need for a seventh. In the United States, where X-ray therapy is not a specialty in itself, practically every practicing radiologist conducts both a diagnostic X-ray unit and an X-ray therapy service.

There are thus literally hundreds of such units in our country, most of which were established without regard to the total national need.

We see only too often a superspecialist in a suburban hospital using special equipment, purchased at great expense by the local community, attempting to carry out an unusual procedure that can be more safely and effectively performed in the nearby urban medical center. Local pride and individual initiative are laudable virtues but they must not cost the life or health of the patient. A superspecialist may provide irreplaceable lifesaving care. But relatively few patients will need his help. He must serve a large population if his knowledge is to continue to grow and his skills are to be kept at peak efficiency. We see that staffing every hospital with a complete roster of superspecialists could be harmful.

Our general hospitals, devoted mainly to the care of acute, short-term illness, are symptomatic of the episodic nature and lack of continuity that pervades our medical care. Moreover, the discharge of chronically ill patients from the general hospital to the miserably inadequate care in nursing homes re-emphasizes our lack of real concern for the chronically ill and the aged.

Institutions for the Chronically Ill

Chronic disease care is the shame of modern medicine. General hospitals do not provide long-term care except for an occasional wealthy patient who can afford the large per diem costs in the private pavilion. General hospitals welcome chronically ill patients only for the treatment of acute episodes and for important complications. After the emergency is over, general hospitals accept little or no responsibility for those needing continued institutional care.

The lack of facilities for patients with chronic illness has been pointed up by the Medicare program. Practically all chronically ill patients who can afford institutional care and those medically indigent persons who receive direct governmental payments are sent after discharge from the general hospital to marginal quasi-medical institutions called nursing homes. Most nursing homes are located in renovated large residences not originally designed as medical facilities, and almost one half of them have no nurses. Indeed, according to the National Nursing Home Survey of 1957,[12] about 40 per cent of all licensed nursing homes, in spite of the name, had not a single professional or practical nurse on the staff. Practically none had an attending physician. Half of the patients in nursing homes had been seen by a physician at least once during the previous month, but one fifth of all nursing home patients had not been

[12] Jerry Solen, D. W. Roberts, D. E. Kreuger, Anna Mae Baney, *Nursing Homes—Their Patients and Care* (Washington, D. C.: U.S. Government Printing Office, 1957).

visited even once by a physician for at least six months, and one out of six had not received medical attention for at least a year.

Even with the upgrading improvement implicit in Medicare approval, our institutions for the chronically ill provide such a sharp contrast with facilities for patients with acute illnesses that future historians may well compare the care they provide with that given by primitive tribes who sent their aged and chronically ill out of the village to fend for themselves. Moreover, even if an adequate skeleton medical staff could be recruited, there would be an unjustifiable waste of physicians' time. Practicing physicians are not likely to be willing to spend their valuable time waiting for traffic lights to turn green as they drive all over town or out into the country among many small scattered nursing homes to care for their patients.

Institutions for the Mentally Ill

The sad plight of patients in the isolated mental disease hospital is depressing. Separate custodial institutions euphemistically called "hospitals for the mentally ill" document the isolation of psychiatry. They will continue to provide primitive care as long as they remain outside the mainstream of medicine. Most such institutions now lack, among other things, a resident staff, an active roster of general physicians, specialists, nurses, and, above all, psychiatrists. To be sure, remote custodial institutions do not attract professional personnel. But most newly fledged psychiatrists prefer to be concerned with a very few patients with relatively minor psychiatric illness rather than devote themselves to a large number with serious mental disease.

Economic Differences

The contrast between voluntary and municipal hospitals punctuates the differences in medical care by economic level. Indeed, since Medicare, and the pressures to provide a modicum of decent medical care to the slum dwellers of our large cities, the role and function of the municipal hospital are now being re-examined. On the other hand, the gradual decrease in the number of proprietary hospitals, that is, privately owned hospitals run like a business for profit, augurs well for an improvement in the quality of medical care.

Beacons to the Future

Most important of all, those individual hospitals scattered throughout our country that have a long tradition of practicing the best medicine primarily for the benefit of the patient stand out as beacons to guide us to the medical care of the future. To be sure, in recent years complicated internal problems of hospital efficiency have cropped up, and must be solved if the great hospitals of our country are to continue to provide leadership.

We may go one step further. If we reorganize and

strengthen our hospitals, total medical care must improve. This is not to say that reorganization can be done entirely within the walls of the hospital. Each change will reverberate in our communities and affect professional, social, and economic relationships in medical care.

Preventive Medicine

There has been an artificial and forced separation between preventive and curative medicine in our country. Modern preventive medicine is concerned not only with the prevention of disease but with the prevention of disability and the postponement of untimely death. Preventive medicine, for many years a tool of the public health officer, is now also an integral part of clinical medicine for the individual patient. Moreover, the science of epidemiology — the study of all the factors that affect the occurrence and course of illness — can now be helpful in diagnosis as it has been in the prevention of the spread of disease in the past. Thus, if the patient coughing up blood is a heavy cigarette smoker, the known epidemiologic association between cigarette smoking and lung cancer calls attention to the diagnostician that there is an increased probability that the bleeding is caused by cancer rather than, for example, tuberculosis. Another useful epidemiologic guide to diagnosis is a history of occupational exposure, for example, that of the house painter to lead or the coal miner to rock dust.

Prevention of infectious disease by vaccination or by providing preventive advice to a patient planning to travel to an underdeveloped country is obvious. But, accumulating medical knowledge has blurred and is now obliterating the line between preventive and curative medicine. The biochemist is identifying the predisposing chemical basis for more and more illnesses so that prevention can now be applied to noninfectious disease. An example is the search in all newborn babies for phenylketonuria to prevent mental deficiency. Individual medical procedures may encompass both prevention and treatment, for example, in the complete care of the patient with chronic disease to include prevention of complications, deformity, or disability and vocational guidance and rehabilitation.

Medical Standards

Medical standards have been slow in evolving. Reverence for the physician and the belief that he was all wise was a standard in itself. This attitude has been expressed through the confidential physician-patient relationship that has been so valuable in the solution of intimate medical problems. But within this relationship the physician, in Dr. George Mackenzie's phrase, after greeting his patient closed the door of his office to the outside world, which in turn made his medical decision final and immutable. It is no surprise that the physician loudly complains when others, in proposing standards, will in effect look over his shoulder as he cares for his patient. This point of view is reinforced by the threat to the physician of malpractice suits. This whole matter is further complicated by the inability of the average patient to judge the quality of medical care he receives from his physician.

In spite of these attitudes, a few medical standards have been established. These include environmental standards, for example, in the structure of a hospital to prevent the patient from being burned to death in a fire or to keep to a minimum the spread of infection. Criteria have been established for the diagnosis of certain illnesses, including diseases of the heart, rheumatic fever, and rheumatoid arthritis. As a protection to the patient, the Commission on Hospital Accreditation has required that a hospital committee review the examination of all tissue specimens removed by the surgeon to validate the need for the operation. There are, however, no comparable standards established to verify a medical diagnosis. All of the existing standards tend to be piecemeal and to be peripheral to what the physician actually does when he cares for a patient.

But the situation is now changed. The explosion of medical knowledge and increasing specialization now make it unreasonable to believe that any doctor can possibly know enough to make a final decision on every problem presented to him. Thus, the inevitable pressures have created an inescapable need for a precise set of medical standards to serve as a reference point in evaluating the quality of medical practice. Such standards must reflect not only the maximum benefits of modern medical knowledge, skills, and facilities that could be supplied to the patient; indeed, such standards should summarize the best present-day medical care and be constantly modified to conform with advances in medical progress.

The definition of precise medical standards might appear at first glance to be an impossible task. But actual experience in the Department of Preventive Medicine at the Harvard Medical School over the past twenty years has demonstrated their feasibility. Indeed, they are defined and redefined each year by our fourth-year students as they conduct a health resources survey of a community.

In making the survey, each student is asked to imagine that he has just completed his formal period of medical education and has entered into practice in the community of his choice. He is given the case histories of four seriously ill patients who seek his help (see the Appendix). The case histories are selected so as to cover the range of all commonly used medical resources extending from the availability of a qualified consultant or a special laboratory test in a highly specialized field of medicine through the use of an acute hospital, chronic hospital, or nursing home to ancillary medical skills such as physiotherapy, public health nursing, and medical social service. The survey also includes all of the economic and social facilities that might be needed to give the patient complete medical care.

The student's first task is to prepare a set of medical standards upon which the optimal care of his patients will be based. These standards represent the best of existing scientific knowledge, medical skills, and medical and social resources. This set of optimum resources is then used as the reference point against which he will measure the actual facilities found in the community of his choice. Such standards have universal application, because they represent the best that can be done. He then goes to this community, assumes that he is the responsible physician, and collects and records quantitative and qualitative information about the medical personnel, institutions, facilities, and services available for the care of his four patients. These data on existing facilities and services are compared with his set of standards. The student notes the differences between the optimal and actual resources. Obviously the "gap" between optimal standards and actual practice will be greater in the medically less well developed areas. But in any area, the closing of this gap represents the job that remains to be done. The student then makes practical recommendations for the care of "his four patients," for the repair of the deficiencies, and for the improvement of the quality of medical care in the community.

After reviewing thousands of such reports collected since 1947, it is clear that an intelligent medical student can identify the possible benefits that could be brought to the patient through the maximum use of medical knowledge, physicians' services, specialized skills, and laboratory, institutional, and social facilities.

In the future, the medical schools, already responsible for many other kinds of standards in medicine, working together with the medical profession acting through its general and specialty organizations, will have to establish definitive standards of medical practice. If they do not, governmental agencies and others concerned with the development of medical care programs will by default be forced by their needs to create medical standards of their own.

With a precise set of standards for medical care and data on medical needs and resources, operations research can aid in the development of a more efficient system of medical care.

The Impact of Contemporary
Technology and Automation

The impact of contemporary technology and automation on medicine can be clearly seen, for example, in the development of machines physically attached to and immediately concerned with the life or health of the patient. These may be in the form of an artificial organ such as a kidney or heart, a feedback (servo) mechanism to control blood pressure or other human physiological functions, an electronic prosthesis to help paraplegic patients to walk, or a sensory aid to help the blind to read.

In analyzing the impact of contemporary technology and automation on medicine, my observations are limited to those general principles governing the most effective application of machines in the preservation of health, the prevention and treatment of disease and disability, and the postponement of untimely death. The actual design, the detailed structure, and the mechanism of the operation of the machines are the concern and within the competence of the engineer and will not be treated here.

The availability of machines to support or replace the function of a diseased vital organ or re-establish the equilibrium of a disturbed physiologic system creates two new problems that must be resolved if the potential medical benefits of automation and technology are to be realized. The first involves the compatibility of man and machine, and the second concerns the ethical conflicts precipitated by the man-machine interaction. The solution of these two problems is fundamental to all planning.

Compatibility of Man and Machine

The basic question of compatibility of man and machine must be resolved by the engineer and the physician working together. A machine may perform beautifully at its assigned task but may, at the same time, harm or even kill the patient. An artificial heart may pump blood effectively but may also damage the blood cells or cause clotting within the patient's blood vessels. Such incompatibilities become even more threatening when more than one machine is hooked up to the patient at the same time. In the future, a patient in shock may be treated with both an artificial heart and an artificial lung to tide him over an acute episode, and the safety of this combined operation must be assured.

Collaboration between engineer and physician is a *sine qua non* if machines are to help patients. Once collaboration has begun, there must be almost continuous feedback in both directions to maintain the equilibrium so essential if each is to make his best contribution to the most effective solution of the problem. Physicians and engineers must also work together in establishing standards for the design, installation, and maintenance of machines taking over important physiological functions. Indeed, standards governing such devices must assure the same level of quality control as those now guiding the testing of new drugs for effectiveness and for lack of harmful effects.

Ethical Considerations
A New Principle of Treatment
Devices that are attached to patients and may have an immediate effect on their life or health introduce a new principle of medical treatment. In the past, treatment of patients has been directed primarily toward supporting normal physiologic functions. Medical treatment eliminated dangerous invaders, as the streptococcus is eliminated with penicillin; boosts the function of an organ, as digitalis does for the heart; replaces a deficient vital substance, as insulin does in a diabetic patient; or relieves symptoms, as aspirin does for a headache. The surgeon's task has been one of removal or repair. He excises such noxious foci as an inflamed appendix or a cancerous tumor; removes an obstructive mass such as an enlarged prostate; reforms a maldeveloped structure such as that in congenital heart disease; or replaces worn-out tissue, as in the case of a badly damaged arthritic joint.

But now modern technology permits us to replace vital organ function with mechanical devices. Failure can result in disaster. The tragedy of the malfunction of substitute organs is dramatic and imposes serious obligations upon the engineer, the manufacturer, the hospital, the surgeon, the medical and maintenance staff, and the service personnel.

There is one historical precedent that focuses the practical and ethical problems for us. During polio epidemics, patients suffering permanent paralysis of the muscles of breathing could be kept alive for many years by the artificial respirator, and the wire carrying electric current to the respirator became the patient's lifeline. The need for perpetual intensive care of these helpless patients hung like a pall over the hospital ward, and elaborate precautions were instituted to safeguard the patient in the event of power or respirator failure. The ethical question of terminating treatment never really arose, because polio epidemics were uncommon, severely paralyzed patients relatively few, the number of respirators adequate, and most of the patients children with their lives ahead of them.

Now the prospect is different. We are not concerned with a few paralyzed survivors of an epidemic but with hoards of patients ceaselessly seeking replacement for their worn-out organs. We are not faced with bringing life-long care to a few children but to adults, most of them elderly, who have exhausted such vital functions as those of heart or kidney.

We must examine this imminent situation most carefully because of the inevitable conflicts governing life and death within the mores of our society. The ethical considerations are many: establishment of lists governing priority of installation; financing to obviate economic and social discrimination so that ability to pay may not become the criterion of eligibility; and preparation of guidelines, if indeed any are possible, for decisions as to overt termination of treatment.

Lifesaving Machines

Let us begin with those wonderful, most favorable situations where the machine can be lifesaving instead of life-preserving, and where the many difficult problems of lifelong treatment do not arise. There are excellent examples where a short period of treatment with the machine could save the patient's life. We can turn again to the past when there were many patients with mild poliomyelitis who suffered only temporary paralysis of their respiratory muscles and were kept alive, often brought to complete recovery, by the artificial respirator.

A modern example is the artificial kidney. The patient whose urine output has suddenly been shut down because of acute mercury poisoning, or as a result of an improperly matched transfusion, will survive with normal kidney function if the artificial kidney can take over for the few weeks required to heal these vital organs.

In the future we may look forward to similar situations with the artificial heart. Death may result from the temporary inability of the heart to deliver enough blood to vital organs, as in the case of the previously healthy man struck down by a severe heart attack or the young person suffering from an overwhelming infection not amenable to antibiotic treatment. Such patients might survive in the future if a "booster heart" were plugged in to carry the circulation until normal defenses and healing mechanisms could control the acute illness. Indeed, lives are already being saved by the cardiac pacemaker when, in severe heart attacks, death is threatened by disturbances in heart rhythm.

Requirements do not loom large in such temporary lifesaving situations but even here they must be satisfied. No waiting list is possible. The emergency devices must be immediately available. Devices once designed should not be difficult to manufacture and should be in sufficient supply. But the limited number and spotty distribution of surgeons qualified to implant the machines will in our present system of medical care pose grave problems.

The cost of temporary devices and their installation and maintenance may well be too great for the large majority of those who might be benefited. But it is likely that voluntary and private health insurance agencies can insure against the relatively predictable costs of temporary devices. This is in marked contrast with permanent devices, where a guarantee of large sums of governmental funds will be necessary to assure their prolonged operation. Moreover, in the use of temporary devices we are not faced with decisions as to overt termination of treatment, because treatment can be stopped when the patient recovers from his acute disease.

Life-Preserving Machines

When lifelong treatment becomes necessary, we face a new set of ethical problems. But we can take advantage of one fact. Ethical problems are less critical with plug-in devices that supplement function than with permanent machines that replace vital organs. In the case of the artificial heart, so long as the patient's own heart is not removed during the operation, the ethics of installation and maintenance of heart boosters are similar to those already governing the use of the heart pacemaker.

But when it becomes necessary to remove the patient's heart, place it on the table, and implant a complete mechanical replacement, ethical considerations loom large. The patient's life is dependent entirely on the uninterrupted and effective performance of the substitute heart. Automatic safety devices to provide further safeguards to the patient are essential, but their use will in turn create new ethical issues: the patient's geographic accessibility to follow-up care will weigh very heavily in the decision to insert a permanent cardiac replacement. But whatever the circumstances, the surgeon and the engineer will carry heavy ethical responsibilities for assuring maximum protection of the patient before complete cardiac replacement is attempted.

Overt Termination of Treatment

A decision as to overt termination of treatment conflicts sharply with our ethic that euthanasia by a positive act, that is, an act of commission, is forbidden. We do not accept the idea that the life of an aged, senile, helpless individual may be terminated by injecting air into his veins. On the other hand, euthanasia by an act of omission is usually tolerated. Chronically ill, deteriorating patients with a clearly diagnosed, painful, fatal illness are often kept comfortable and quiet with large doses of analgesics and sedatives. Such treatment decreases the patient's intake of food, and the occurrence of a terminal illness such as bronchopneumonia becomes more likely.

Situations must eventually develop where a productive patient's life can be continued only with the use of a permanent machine. It is at this point that the full weight of all of the ethical considerations of priority lists, adequate financing, and decisions as to overt termination of treatment will become most difficult.

The crucial decision as to overt termination of treatment, under such circumstances, can be focused by the probable course of many patients. Let us imagine that a permanent artificial device was installed when the patient was a productive citizen and that it kept him alive until he became senile, when he was unaware of his surroundings and unable to perform at the simplest level. His permanent device had completely replaced the function of his own heart. Regardless of his deteriorated state, it would be simply impossible to turn off the artificial heart as long as we adhered to our present ethic.

When permanent devices permitting ambulation of the patient are developed, new practical and legal problems will be created. In the case of the artificial heart. these will include such questions as his eligibility for an automobile driver's license, benefits from workmen's compensation, or the permission for the patient to enter into occupations where sudden failure of his artificial heart might threaten his own safety or that of others.

The Time Is Now

The final answers to all such questions must depend upon the nature and the reliability of the particular kind of artificial organ. Careful and thorough consideration must be given to each kind of machine as soon as development has proceeded to the point where the final product may be visualized. Indeed, the development of the artificial heart, as an example, has already gone far enough; it is now the responsibility of government through the National Science Foundation or the Department of Health, Education, and Welfare, or of a large private foundation, to bring together engineers, physicians, theologians, psychologists, lawyers, and other lay leaders to establish a set of ethics and standards governing the implantation and use of the organ and decisions as to termination of treatment.

Interaction between Doctor and Machine

Now we turn to a set of machines the primary impact of which is to help the physician practice his profession. These include measuring devices as used in automated laboratory tests, monitoring equipment as used in intensive care units, and analytic instrumentation to aid the physician in such processes as medical diagnosis. Let us examine the principles that govern the interaction between doctor and machine. No machine can replace the physician but it can relieve him of those tasks that it performs at least as effectively as he does.

We must begin by identifying those physicians' tasks that can be performed as effectively by a machine. In doing so, the assessment of the effectiveness of the machine must be made primarily in terms of patient benefit. It may be considered adequate if it performs a specific task with at least the same benefit to the patient and yet saves enough time for the doctor (or other paramedical personnel) to justify its original and operating costs. But, regardless of the effectiveness with which the machine performs the allocated task, the patient must not fare worse than he would have if the machine had not been used.

In essence, the allocation of physicians' tasks to a machine follows the same principles previously laid down for allocating physicians' tasks to ancillary medical personnel. Indeed, when both of these steps have been completed, operations research theory must be applied to obtain the best balance between physician, ancillary medical personnel, and machine in carrying out specific medical functions.

There is another important principle. The machine must not be interposed between the patient and his physician nor be used as an excuse for not providing him with the attention and time of the physician. Even the best balanced medical care system is unsatisfactory if it does not meet the personal needs of the patient. In my view, the personal evaluation of the patient and his guidance and reassurance by his physician (and by other medical personnel) must continue to be a major attribute of medical care. Indeed, any successful system of medical care interrelating the activities of physicians, other medical personnel, and machines must have as *the* essential ingredient "tender loving care."

Machines Can Be Helpful

Computer-controlled automated counting and measuring equipment has many applications to medicine, as is best illustrated by examples in the hospital. Most obvious are the machine-aided management functions of accounting, personnel efficiency, and the transportation and messenger systems adapted from industry. Inventory control can be effective in avoiding food waste in the hospital kitchen; it is precise enough to maintain an adequate stock of essential drugs in the pharmacy and to keep a count of the appropriate number of units of all of the types of blood in the blood bank.

Specific medical management functions can also be facilitated by machines. Procedures such as those for the admission and discharge of hospital patients and the retrieval of information from medical records when casually performed, as they are in many hospitals, breed much dissatisfaction from patients and from physicians. Using appropriate machine-aided management functions, the hospital admission procedure should not delay the treatment of the anxious patient nor the relief of his symptoms while he and his family recite the identifying and financial information so close to the hearts of hospital administrators. Similarly, medical record information could become immediately available to the physician for guidance in treatment of his patients at all times of the day and night.

More important, there are hospital procedures that prove to be much more complicated than we might suspect and where human error may seriously affect the course of the patient and his disease. Examples are the administration of drugs and laboratory testing.

The patient must receive his prescribed medication in the exact dose at the precise time. There is a chain of events subject to human error all along the way from the moment the physician writes his prescription until the patient receives his medication. Except in the case of ordinary drugs such as aspirin, the nurse must request the prescribed drug in precise dosage from the pharmacy; the pharmacist must check the prescribed dosage for efficiency and toxicity; he must have the drug in stock; and the prescription must be filled correctly.

The bottle of medicine has to be delivered promptly to the appropriate nursing station, and the nurse must give the drug to the patient at the proper time. She must make certain that he swallows it and she must keep an eye on the patient to observe the desired response or toxic effects. There must be a record available to the physician specifying the dose of the drug, the time of the administration, and the results. Many different automated "quality control" schemes are now under study to protect the patient against all of these possible sources of human error in drug administration.

Laboratory testing is subject to similar kinds of errors, which may be kept at a minimum with the assistance of machines. The information passed from the physician through the nurse to the laboratory in the form of an order, and returned to him in an accurate and timely report of the test, must be reliable. But there is, all along the line, a chain of possible human errors in the collection of the specimen, the tubes that may be lost, broken, or mislabeled, the technical mistakes in the laboratory, and the mistakes in recording and reporting the results of the test to the physician. Here again, technological knowledge to solve the problem is available, and machine-aided control systems are being rapidly developed. And again by these examples we are reminded that the purpose of automation and the application of technology to medicine is to benefit the patient.

Saving the Physician's Time

The scarcest and most valuable commodity in the medicine of the future will be the time of the physician. We have already pointed out how tasks that do not demand his background, education, knowledge, skills, and experience may be delegated to other medical professional or vocational workers or to machines. Now we must examine the ways in which those tasks that do demand the physician's time and his competence may be performed more effectively by him with the aid of analytical instrumentation. Let us use diagnosis of disease as an example.

Diagnosis is a task that properly demands a great deal of a physician's time, because it is a major function that he cannot delegate to others. Recently a great deal of attention has been given to the role of automation and the electronic computer in medical diagnosis. Unfortunately, much unnecessary confusion has been created by the extravagant claims that machines will replace the physician in diagnosis. If, instead, diagnosis is considered as a form of pattern analysis, both the computer and automation can be helpful to him in many specific ways in the diagnosis of disease.

The manifestations making up a pattern of illness include the symptoms revealed by the history, the signs of illness disclosed by physical examination, and the abnormal results of laboratory and other tests. The various manifestations of illness — symptoms, signs, and test results — vary in their adaptability to the computer. Laboratory and other test results, usually in the form of numbers, can easily be handled by the computer. In contrast, responses to questions in the history and signs revealed by physical examination have to be purposely sought out by the physician, are less easy to quantify, and require professional interpretation. When a physician makes a diagnosis, he seeks out the manifestations of the illness by history, physical examination, and laboratory tests, arranges them in a pattern, and compares this with the patterns of illness stored in his memory. In a simple case he selects the pattern in his memory that most closely corresponds to that of the patient and applies its name to the patient's illness. In the case of the child with fever, a running nose, blurry eyes, and a blotchy rash, who had been exposed to his brother with a similar illness two weeks before, the physician fits these facts into a pattern, compares it with the patterns in his memory, and calls it measles.

Often, however, the diagnosis is more difficult, because the patient's illness may correspond to patterns of many different diseases. The physician then makes a number of tentative diagnoses and seeks out additional manifestations of the patient's illness, for example, by laboratory testing that may distinguish between them. The physician may not be able to tell whether the patient with pain in his right upper abdomen and nausea, vomiting, and constipation has an ulcer of the stomach or duodenum or has gall bladder disease. He orders X rays of the upper gastrointestinal tract and of the gall bladder, and with such additional information he may be able to decide whether the patient has one of the two illnesses or a third that he had not previously considered.

A good diagnostician performs all of these steps with precision. To maintain his competence he consults medical publications, and he checks his performance by following the course of disease in his patients. He also rearranges his memory patterns as newly recognized diseases are identified and as additional information becomes available on previously known illnesses.

If the physician is to be assisted by the computer in diagnosis, he must take advantage of its speed, the reliability and capacity of its memory bank, and its precision in the matching of patterns. For example, the computer can aid the physician in solving some of his undiagnosed cases by supplying a "printout" of a list of all the diseases compatible with the patient's symptoms, signs, and test results thus reminding him of diseases he may not have considered.

Laboratory Tests

In the future, most laboratory tests will be performed by automated machines and the data processed by the computer. Laboratory measurements, usually in the form of numbers, for example, of the blood sugar, or electronic records such as electrocardiograms, can easily be handled. The computer will also recognize and count patterns such as those of the blood cells or of the chromosomes. As we have already noted, the computer can decrease human errors in the processing of the tests. Moreover, the computer will automatically request the physician to repeat unsatisfactory tests, for example, when the tube containing the specimen is lost, broken, or mislabeled; when the pattern of the results of a specific test on a particular day is out of line; or when the testing equipment breaks down.

Physical Examinations

In contrast to automated test results, practically all findings on physical examination must be sought individually and usually require interpretation by the physician. For example, the sounds and murmurs of the heart may be recorded on tape and interpreted automatically by the computer. But the proper placing of the microphone on the chest to pick up the heart tones at appropriate locations first requires that a physician listen to the heart with a stethoscope exactly as he does when he performs a physical examination. To be sure, an automated test procedure may be devised to replace specific steps in the physical examination, for example, measuring the size of the heart by X ray. All in all, replacement of the physician's examination by automatic methods would require a revolutionary approach that is not yet discernible. The computer will not soon replace the physician in the physical examination of the patient.

There is also a grave danger in the automation of the physical examination which must be guarded against. Very simple procedures, such as the inspection of the patient by the physician, now yield information essential to precise diagnosis. As far as I am aware, no claims have yet been made that the computer will survey the patient and say, "he looks sick." In our zeal to automate medical care and to design more objective measuring devices, we must make a conscious effort not to discard simple useful methods, not now adaptable to the machine, that provide crucial information.

Medical History

The medical history is the key to diagnosis. Because history taking is so time consuming many efforts have been made in the past to delegate this responsibility to a nurse or to the patient himself by questionnaire. These efforts have been largely unsuccessful. Of all medical procedures, history taking makes the greatest demands on the physician's knowledge, ingenuity, experience, training, and understanding of disease. Medical history taking is not a random process. Instead, as your physician focuses down on or rules out a diagnosis, his lines of questioning depend on the nature of your illness and your responses. In effect, he fits together a long series of short interlocking questionnaires. As he questions you, the good diagnostician asks the pertinent questions and does not waste time with irrelevant ones. He also keeps an open mind so that if the "pertinent" line of reasoning is not fruitful, he may explore other possibilities.

As your history is being taken, your answers will depend upon your understanding, intelligence, reliability, and mental state. Your physician, to be certain of your exact complaints, often asks you the same question in a number of different ways. Moreover, precisely the same response may have more serious significance in one patient than in another. Indeed, the "sick headache" of a nervous, middle-aged woman without serious illness may be described in more vivid terms than may the headache due to a brain tumor in a stoic patient. History taking as now practiced is far from being amenable to programming on a computer. It should be a fertile field for research.

Research on the Diagnostic Process

We have seen a limited number of ways in which the machine may aid the physician in diagnosis in our present system of medical practice. It will become clear in the "Plan for the Medicine of the Future" from the extrapolation of our research that the structure of medical practice itself must be modified for the more effective use of automated instrumentation in saving the physician's time.

One of my colleagues, Professor Murray Eden, suggested a study design that has yielded information relevant to better doctor-machine interaction in medical diagnosis. In asking the question, How does a doctor make a diagnosis? he proposed that a number of physicians be tested with a series of case histories all with the same chief complaint. Professor Eden, Dr. William Kannel, and I selected as the chief complaint "pain in the chest," because it occurs in a wide variety of diseases most of which are diagnosable. The physician being tested was to be given a brief description of the patient, for example, that she was a twenty-four-year-old white, Irish housewife with pain in the right upper chest of two days duration, following which he was permitted to ask the patient[1] any question he wished provided that he told us the differential diagnosis that provoked it.

It soon became evident that the test physicians fell into one of three categories. On the one hand there were

[1] As we sat around the table with the physician under test, Dr. William Kannel who had written up the case histories acted as the patient, Professor Eden kept a record of the "logic tree" of the physician's reasoning for computer analysis, and I followed the changing differential diagnosis as the questioning proceeded.

those who followed faithfully the order of history taking they had learned as second-year medical students. At the other extreme were those who asked a few questions, settled on a diagnosis, and spent the rest of the time defending it. In between was the large group of physicians who, with varying degrees of skill, followed tentative lines of reasoning until they arrived at the diagnosis.

The test physician sometimes asked the key question very early and arrived at a definitive diagnosis within a few minutes. We could not tell whether he was "smart" or just "lucky." We were then faced with the unattractive prospect of doing a long, statistical study on each physician to find out exactly how he made a diagnosis.

Then we realized that we were asking the wrong question. More relevant to precise diagnosis than the order of questioning is the identification of those key questions whose answers immediately reveal the diagnosis. Looking back over our records, we discovered what we should have known, that in cases in which pain in the chest was the chief complaint the question which most often revealed the diagnosis was, "What did the chest film show?" The second most revealing question, particularly in older adults, was, "What about the electrocardiogram?"

Many patients are admitted to the hospital in the afternoon. Unless a physician writes an emergency order, the chest X ray of the patient admitted with pain in the chest is taken the next morning and reported later that day or on the second morning. Thus, in the usual course of events, the most important datum on the patient does not have adequate priority. To be sure, in emergency cases many useful short cuts are introduced by the examining physician. But these tend to be *ad hoc* decisions of the particular physician on duty and have not been systematically studied. It would seem reasonable that our present method of admission of patients to hospital should be re-examined. In the "Plan for the Medicine of the Future" we shall explore ways in which machine-aided diagnosis may make the hospital admission procedure more efficient.

Impact of Automation and Technology on Research

During the past few decades, under the guidance of the engineer, we have seen the prolific development of all kinds of essential measuring instruments for biological and medical research. But there has been a lag. Machines that measure things were developed at a faster rate than machines to handle the data they produced. Now we are beginning to catch up. Electronic computers now analyze research data at a rate far in excess of our ability to collect them. Moreover, devices are being developed that collect analytical data in a form easily handled by the computer.

In our own laboratory we have recently been blessed

with such a device.[2] In research on human atherosclerosis, the disease responsible for "heart attacks," we have been studying the ways in which fatty substances go in and out of cells from the lining of human blood vessels. All fats have as part of their structure one or many members of a large family of compounds called fatty acids, some saturated and some unsaturated. Identification of these acids in their many compounds is made by a machine called a gas-liquid chromatograph. In each analysis this machine traces a record on paper with a pen in the form of a series of peaks, each representing a different fatty acid, and all rising from a common base line. Until recently we have employed medical students to work at night, painstakingly measuring the size of the peaks, which indicate the relative amount of each fatty acid present in the sample. Now the medical students may spend their time in a more useful way. Calculations are now automatic. The output of the machine is transmitted through a pair of telephone wires to an electronic laboratory, where it is recorded on tape and fed into a computer, which then "prints out" the proportionate amount of each fatty acid present in each sample. Our experimental results are immediately available and we have eliminated the "million monkey method" of handling our research data.

[2] William Simon, William P. Castelli, and David D. Rutstein, "Semi-Automatic Remote Gas-Liquid Chromatographic Analysis," *The Journal of Gas Chromotography*, forthcoming, 1967.

Machines can also be helpful in research in a more fundamental way, that is, in the design of experiments. With increasing specialization, problems are necessarily studied in depth. But studies in depth, almost by their very nature, demand a narrow approach. As a result, many of the great recent accessions to medical knowledge have been studied in carefully controlled simplified systems where individual variables may be precisely measured. But an event occurring in such an artificial system may not reflect the actual mechanism in the more complex intact animal.

In his search for "basic knowledge" the research specialist has moved away seriatim from the organ system in the intact animal to the isolated organ, to the single cell, the cellular elements, the molecular groupings, down through chemical reactions to the individual molecule, and finally, to the growing family of tiny particles where mass and energy become one. Indeed, the research scientist has often become so fascinated with his studies of such progressively disintegrated systems that he may forget the complex organism — man — that started him on his way. This is understandable because the scientist tends to continue to explore the research system in which he has been successful. But the fact remains that, to determine whether new discoveries in isolated systems are relevant to the patient, a whole new series of reintegrating studies in more complex systems are necessary, progressing seriatim in the opposite direction, from the simplified system to the intact animal and to man. Unfortunately, this stage of investigation has become relatively neglected.

But now we can take advantage of a new approach. The processing of data is no longer the limiting factor. Now that data-handling equipment and processing have caught up with methods and devices for the collection of data, and the on-line electronic computer now permits the simultaneous measurement of many variables in more complex physiological systems of single organs or the intact animal, we may more effectively design our medical and biological experiments. This does not mean that we should give up our present methods of study in isolated systems. They have revealed important knowledge with broad biological significance that must be continued and expanded. At the same time, it is imperative that the way we design experiments be intensively studied to take advantage of contemporary technology.

Practical Examples of New Research Design
Total Organ Function

The advantages of this new approach can be illustrated by studies of the total function of the kidney. Kidney function is complex and involves many variables, among which are all of the substances entering from the bloodstream via the renal artery and returned to the bloodstream via the renal vein, the compounds excreted into the urine, and the dynamic changes in blood flow through the kidney. Present studies of this organ tend to be limited to single aspects in which a few variables are measured at a time, with disjointed results when one attempts to relate one experiment to another. Moreover, the present method of study makes it difficult, if not impossible, to evaluate the interdependence of all of the variables — which in essence is total kidney function.

It is now possible to design experiments in which most of the important functions of the kidney could be measured simultaneously and their interrelationships defined and analyzed by the electronic computer. Such research should simplify the diagnosis of kidney disease in an individual case, because the independent variables would be identified and it would no longer be necessary to measure the dependent ones. More important, this line of investigation will undoubtedly lead to a better understanding of the total function of this important complex organ. With such data we could also simulate total kidney function on the computer. Such research on total organ function has the great advantage that it is both basic and applied.

Better Epidemiologic Studies

As another example, we may now perform more comprehensive epidemiologic studies of disease in the human population. Epidemiology is the science concerned with the study of all of the factors that affect the occurrence, distribution, and course of disease in a population. Many factors are obviously involved. In infectious disease these include the presence and the nature of the external invader, such as a germ, the channels — air, water, milk, or insect bite — through which it reaches the victim, and the characteristics of the host, including his age, sex, genetic background, and previous illnesses and immunizations that affect his resistance.

But epidemiology is not limited to the study of infectious disease. Its greatest present use is in developing leads to unravel the mechanism of diseases of unknown cause. In the 1940's, the exploding epidemic of lung cancer and its epidemiologic association with cigarette smoking started the intensive research on the constituents of cigarette smoke responsible for converting normal tissue into cancer of the lung. In the future, the greatest potential contribution of epidemiology is to reveal leads to disentangle the many variables that may interact in the mechanism of such diseases of unknown cause as psychiatric illness.

It is clear that the impact of contemporary automation and technology permitting many variables to be studied simultaneously will revolutionize medical research and hasten the growth of medical knowledge.

An Ever-Present Danger

There is a danger to be guarded against in the increasing use of complicated machines in medical research. Some of our preclinical investigators and research physicians tend to spend less and less time in understanding science as an inductive method of reasoning and more and more time in learning how to operate increasingly complicated equipment. Too often young investigators become married to an esoteric technique and concentrate on finding ways in which it may be applied in the research laboratory rather than on following their research problem wherever it may lead and using whatever techniques may be indicated. In effect, some of our younger investigators are becoming supertechnicians instead of research scientists. Poorly designed experiments are not worth doing — even with the most elaborate equipment.

Research accomplishment will be greater if the scientist, although completely understanding the function of his machines and knowing how to operate them, will concentrate on the design of his experiments, currently evaluate his data, plan each step along the way, relate his studies to advances in his field — in short, spend more of his time thinking about his problem. He may then delegate to supertechnicians the romantic tasks of manipulating electronics, stainless steel, chromium, and crystal. To be sure, he must stay "close by" and live in his laboratory to take advantage of unexpected and casual observations.

Operations Research Can Help the Investigator

Medical research is becoming ever more complicated and extraordinarily expensive. Individual investigators, because of the need for precise trustworthy measurements, purchase their own equipment and operate it under their own supervision.

The time has come when investigators will have to share some equipment and personnel to keep at a minimum the growing waste that occurs when space, equipment, and other facilities are not fully used. If not, with an eventual ceiling on the proportion of gross national product to be spent on medical research, a significant number of worthy grant requests will go unfunded. Certainly automated computer-controlled laboratory equipment can maintain a high standard of precision on run-of-the-mill tests. There is no reason why a single automated laboratory for such tests should not suffice for each research institution. In any event, there is an urgent need for the application of operations research to determine where the routine aspects of fundamental research may be made more efficient.

The Research Interface between Mathematics, the Physical and Engineering Sciences, and Medicine

This relatively new research interface between mathematics, the physical and engineering sciences, and technology, on the one hand, and medicine and biology, on the other, is pregnant with opportunity. We can visualize the physical and engineering sciences becoming basic to the medicine of the future just as the biochemical sciences have in the recent past. Moreover, we can eagerly look forward to revolutionary, new general biological laws emerging from the introduction of mathematical theory just as world-shaking physical laws have been deduced in the past.

In medicine and biology such research is already under way. The fluid dynamics engineer is now working more closely with investigators of the circulation of the blood. Mathematical theories governing linguistics and communication are providing an added dimension to the study of human behavior. Classical biochemistry is now interwoven with the engineering sciences in research on the mechanism of the synthesis of the protein molecule. Feedback theory is receiving increasing attention in studies of cell function. But such efforts remain piecemeal. There is a lack of scope and continuity in such research because its institutional structure has not yet been developed.

If this new area is to be productive, the medical student must be made aware of its possibilities in his preclinical years. At present, in most medical schools there is no home in any of the departments of preclinical science for the increasing numbers of students with a background in the physical sciences or mathematics who look forward to a career at any of the interfaces between engineering and technology, and medicine. We must find a home for such students so that they will be able to contribute adequately to our national health.

There are many ways to relate these sciences, engineering and mathematics, to biology and medicine and to find a home for the physical science, engineering, and mathematical student entering medical school. New preclinical departments can be established in medical schools; engineering schools could add clinical departments and hospital facilities; or schools of engineering and medicine in the same or different universities could join together in collaboration on research, teaching, and medical care. This last approach would appear to be most practical, although local considerations may dictate other solutions. An example of one operating program is the biomathematical consultation and teaching program conducted by the faculty members of the Massachusetts Institute of Technology in the Department of Preventive Medicine at the Harvard Medical School. This program has demonstrated that joint activities can be developed simultaneously in research, in education, and in the solution of medical care problems. We need intensive experimentation to determine how best to establish effective interrelationships to evolve a common language and to define crucial problems for collaborative investigation.

We have now developed the background against which we may project a plan for the medicine of the future.

A Plan for the Medicine of the Future

The plan for the medicine of the future is a practical one. It will take advantage of current trends and the pressures building up within our medical care system. Where trends are not clear, research studies will be recommended. The plan will be directed toward the solution of long-range problems and not toward such immediate and transient ones as the actuarial soundness of paying physicians on a fee-for-service basis in Medicare (Title XVIII, Part B), or the desirability of the Kerr-Mills means test in the Medicaid program, although some of their long-term implications may appear in the plan.

The plan is in no sense a fixed blueprint of a medical care system — it may not predict what *will* happen. Instead it indicates what *could* happen if we took full advantage of our resources, knowledge, and skills. Whether or not this plan, or details of it, be implemented, one thing is clear. The consequences of not planning well for the future of medicine are too grave to contemplate.

Let me give you a simple outline of the plan. We shall emphasize the need for the regional structure of medical care programs, propose a more effective use of medical manpower, indicate ways in which the physician's time may be more strategically applied, take advantage of rapidly advancing automation and technology, suggest added dimensions for medical research, and recommend a system of medical education to meet future needs.

The reference point for the plan will be a scientifically based set of standards, constantly modified to keep pace with medical progress.[1] In practice, the standards represent the ideal against which to measure the quality and relative effectiveness of a particular program. They also serve as a guide to help us do the best we can with what we have and to keep abreast of advances in medicine as they occur.

Regionalization of Medical Care Services

As our hospitals evolve into centers for community health, incorporating all preventive and curative services, we are faced with a serious dilemma. Not every hospital will be able to provide what every patient needs for the prevention and treatment of his disease. If this dilemma is to be resolved, we cannot build the medical system of the future around self-centered individual hospitals as we do today. Instead, through careful planning and efficient transportation and communication systems we have to weave together all medical facilities and personnel into

[1] David D. Rutstein, "Better Health for Americans: The Need for Standards of Medical Care," *Transactions & Studies of the College of Physicians of Philadelphia*, 29 (1962), 170–178.

regional medical service areas centered upon large teaching hospitals that are affiliated with medical schools.

We in this country have had little experience with such medical organization. The needed information must be collected in precisely designed medical care studies. Fortunately, the necessary research and planning funds have been made available by the enactment of the Heart, Cancer, and Stroke Regional Medical Programs Legislation, which was designed to bring the benefits of modern medicine to all victims of these three major groups of diseases and related illnesses. Since there is so little information with which to plan, one cannot escape the conclusion that the first stage in planning is the establishment of community medical research centers where systematic studies may be designed and conducted.

The research program must have two separate foci — a precise definition of medical needs on the one hand and an inventory of medical care resources on the other — if operations research experts and systems analysts are to design test models. Quality control will depend on the application of a well-designed set of medical standards. For example, in a program for the treatment of coronary heart disease patients, the need might be the number of patients with heart attacks requiring intensive care in a particular time interval; the standards would be the criteria for the equipment, personnel, and operation of an intensive care unit; and the resources, the number of available beds in units meeting these criteria.

Estimates of the Needs

Let us turn first to measuring the needs, using the Regional Medical Program Legislation as our model. We might ask ourselves: How many lives could be saved each year if everything possible were done for sufferers from these diseases? Many optimistic answers were given to this question in legislative hearings, but these were the usual puffery that one expects of proponents of legislation testifying before Congressional Committees — the fact is that nobody knows. But we can find out.[2]

We can identify those whose lives might have been saved with optimal treatment by a thorough study of the circumstances of death in a properly selected sample of fatal illnesses.[3] This established method has yielded life-

[2] The series of studies outlined here were developed together with Dr. Osler L. Peterson and other staff members of the Department of Preventive Medicine and with Professor Gerald Rosenthal of the Department of Economics at Harvard University who are already engaged in collecting such data.

[3] In the case of heart disease, cancer, and stroke, valid estimates may be derived from the random sample of deaths selected through death certificates in a particular geographic area specifying the causes of death listed under the rubrics relative to these diseases in the *International List of Causes of Death*, and supplemented by a random sample of all other death certificates to identify those deaths from heart disease, cancer, and stroke where the causes were not specified by the physician on the death certificate.

saving information in maternal and infant mortality studies in the past.[4] A competent team of medical specialists can determine whether the patient had received all the potential benefits of modern medicine and calculate the proportion of those whose lives might have been saved.

But it is not enough to study the postponement of untimely death. We must also have information on the amount and kinds of nonfatal disease requiring prevention and treatment. The burden of severe illness in a community can be estimated from a study of hospital discharge diagnoses. The impact of mild illness can be best estimated from a population survey. By combining these data with information about deaths, we shall have reliable estimates of community medical needs for planning a regional medical care program.

We also require estimates of economic need. The total cost of hospital and ambulatory care will include the capital costs of buildings and equipment and their depreciation, compensation for personnel employed in and out of institutions, fees paid for physicians' services, adminis-

[4] Helen C. Chase, "International Comparison of Perinatal and Infant Mortality: The United States and Six West European Countries," prepared for the United States Department of Health, Education, and Welfare and presented at the Ninety-Fourth Meeting of the American Public Health Association, San Francisco, Calif., November 3, 1966.

trative expenses of insurance and other prepayment plans, expenditures for public health services including immunizations, and payments for treatment modalities including drugs and prostheses.

Uncommonly used superspecialists' services should be strategically located to cover as large a population as possible. Estimates of their capital and maintenance costs, balanced against the costs of transportation to care in a more remote hospital, would be useful in discouraging the establishment of unnecessary units and would favor the more effective use of such services in a regional system. Even in the absence of regional planning, such estimates are needed when a community hospital, for example, is requested to establish a neurosurgical unit although one already exists in the nearby urban teaching hospital.

These studies on the lives that could be salvaged, the impact of mild and severe illness, and the costs of total and superspecialists' services are representative of the research that must be done to obtain precise estimates of need.

Inventory of Resources

Now we can turn the coin over and outline the kinds of studies needed for an inventory of resources. We may begin by making an inventory of institutional facilities with careful consideration given to their type and quality. Included are such resources as hospital beds, laboratory services, immunization and well-baby clinics located in general hospitals, health departments, sanitaria, and chronic and mental disease institutions located within the region. These facilities will have to be looked at not only for the amount and quality of their services but for the very special nature of their resources, such as the availability of rare types of blood in the blood bank or the automated monitoring equipment in an intensive care unit.

The inventory must also comprise those regional services and facilities provided by national and state agencies located elsewhere. Examples are the services of a state laboratory or mental disease hospital; the resources of a federal narcotic treatment center; the Epidemic Intelligence Service of the Communicable Disease Center of the United States Public Health Service; or the emergency program of a national voluntary agency like the Red Cross.

An inventory of the number and quality of all health and medical, professional, and vocational personnel in the region is essential to planning an area-wide program. In the case of physicians, for example, attention must be paid to their qualifications and experience with particular emphasis on their areas of specialization. Again, personnel affiliated with national, state, and other agencies outside of the region but providing services within it must be included.

The inventory of personnel must take into account geographical distribution within the region. While doing so, studies will have to be made of transportation facilities not only to bring personnel to medical institutions and to the patient but also to transport the patient to prevention and treatment services. Transportation services must be evaluated to determine whether they actually provide for special needs — such as those of patients who are receiving care at distant and relatively scarce superspecialist facilities like a radiation treatment center.

The total financial resources for medical care in the region, and the sources that provide them, have to be identified and related to the exact services that they support. A balance sheet can then be set up matching in realistic fashion the costs and the quality and quantity of services provided. Ultimately, with the availability of standards of medical care and priorities of prevention and treatment services, it could be decided whether the financial resources for health and medical care of the region are being expended wisely. If not, the inventory should supply useful information for reorganization of medical care services.

Whatever studies are finally established to evaluate the needs and resources of a region, a procedure must be set up to keep the information up to date.

Operations Research

When research scientists have the collection of information on needs and resources under way, experts in operations research can begin to build their models. As the two groups keep each other informed of their progress, the studies can be sharpened up and the structure of the models reinforced. As a result of such give and take, a model of an entire regional system or, more probably, that of one of its functions should emerge. An obvious example is a model of the optimal use of superspecialists' services that would be worth testing in actual practice in a community setting.

When practical considerations make such testing impossible, the model may be simulated on a computer to obtain additional evidence on how best to balance the needs and resources so as to provide maximal benefit to the patient. Since the various components of the regional system tend to be synergistic — that is, to be more effective than the sum total of their individual contributions — it would probably be wise to set up at least one "model" region where all possible factors are intensively interrelated. The "model" region could be used both as a demonstration and as a medium of education for the creation of similar regional systems elsewhere. Later, as many such studies are conducted throughout the country, individual regions will be able to learn from the experience of others. All of the regional planning data can then be interpreted in the light of the precise set of medical standards — all for the benefit of the patient.

We Can Begin Now

But we do not have to wait for the research results to pour in to begin building our regional systems of medical care.[5] We may in the interim reap many of the benefits of regionalization.

Let us explore my proposal for a regional system. Its over-all framework may be clearly visualized. The present-day general hospital with its inpatient care and ambulatory services would be the core of the hospital of the future. By the turn of the next century it will have to incorporate all preventive and curative personnel and services and become the center for community health. But the new hospital center will no longer be self-centered; it will be carefully interrelated in a community-wide and regional hospital system to meet the total medical care needs of the individual and the community.

Affiliated with the general hospital and located within its surrounding walls will be specialty hospitals, facilities for the care of the broad spectrum of chronic illness including mental disease, a group-practice unit, a clinical preventive medical service, the local health department, and voluntary health agencies providing direct services to patients.

[5] David D. Rutstein, "At the Turn of the Next Century," Lowell Lecture delivered at the Massachusetts General Hospital on May 15, 1963.

Specialty Hospitals

Specialty hospitals can no longer operate as isolated institutions. Treatment limited entirely to the specialty of the hospital is by definition incomplete. Since complete care requires a general physician, and access to whichever specialist may be needed at the moment, these essential services can most easily be provided if the specialty hospital is geographically adjacent to the general hospital in a hospital center in the regional complex. The adjacent geographic location and the affiliation of the specialty with the general hospital will do more than provide good medical care for its patients. It will in return make highly specialized services available to patients in the hospital center and throughout the regional system.

Care of Chronic Illness

In the future, medical care for the chronically ill, to include all gradations from full-time institutional therapy to ambulatory health care in the community, will be provided within the hospital complex in buildings that are specifically designed for this purpose. The chronic disease unit will of course be a simpler structure than that of the acute general hospital since patients who need more intensive care can be transferred. The close proximity of these institutions will allow for education of interns and resident physicians in both acute and chronic illnesses and will make possible easy consultation with specialists when needed.

Mental Disease Hospitals

In the United States, we are beginning to recognize that we must do away with the isolated mental disease hospital. New mental disease units will be built adjacent to general hospitals so that they will be accessible to the patients, their families, and their physicians. The juxta-position of the mental disease hospital and the general hospital will have other important advantages. It will bring the patient with mental disease in contact with research physicians and with modern medical investigation. The patient will be seen through the eyes of a physician in addition to those of a psychiatrist. Because of closer contact, research workers within the general hospital may become aware of mental disease problems susceptible to immediate solution. Finally, affiliation with a general hospital will facilitate the recruitment of resident staff, nurses, and, hopefully, psychiatrists.

By the turn of the next century, a series of graded psychiatric services will have been developed to meet the needs of each individual patient. Depending upon the needs of the individual patient, these will extend all the way from care in the patient's own home through intermittent ambulatory treatment to part-time and, at the other extreme, full-time hospital care.

The Group Practice Unit

In the hospital of the future, all of the physicians on the staff will comprise a group practice unit, located in the building within the hospital grounds of each of the centers of the region. In the main center of the regional complex, the group practice unit will consist of a complete roster of specialists, all of the general physicians practicing in the immediate area, and ancillary medical personnel. In the community centers, the roster would include the more commonly consulted specialists and all of the general physicians. Location on hospital grounds would conserve the time of the physician as he provides ambulatory care in his office and inpatient treatment on the hospital wards. Ambulatory care will benefit also from the proximity of the extensive armamentarium of equipment, personnel, and other facilities of the inpatient service.

Preventive Medicine in the Hospital

At the turn of the next century, when you or your children are seen by a physician you will be evaluated simultaneously for prevention and for treatment. Pediatricians are already spending more time on prevention, particularly when they care for small babies. Medical care in all fields will be concerned increasingly with prevention to conform with the trends in our accumulating knowledge and to anticipate your medical needs.

Preventive medicine units would be found in the main centers in the regional system and in strategically located community centers. The preventive medical service would provide consultation on such matters as the desirability of immunization under special conditions of exposure or risk, such as polio immunization of pregnant women or influenza immunization for patients with chronic heart or lung disease; or interpret epidemiologic data, for example, in describing a diet for the management of a patient recovering from a coronary heart attack; or develop screening programs for all patients for the detection of the early stages of previously unknown disease that is better treated early than late, for example, carcinoma of the cervix of the uterus; or prevent the spread of disease from hospital to the family and to the community, and vice versa, for example, in recent epidemics of staphylococcal infection.

The evolution ˙ ᶜ the regional hospital system will open the way for an ˁ ˑctiᵛ ᵘnification of preventive and curative services. ᾽he health department will be transferred from its political surroundings in city hall to the professional environment of the hospital center. The function of the health department will be interrelated with those of the therapeutic services through the preventive medical service in activities such as community-wide immunization against disease, for example, polio and measles; interrelating school health services to total medical care as is done so well in Denmark; in prevention and treatment of man-made diseases, for example, those due to toxic agents whether they be in smog, the air of an industrial plant, the dust from an insecticide in the field, the smoke of a cigarette, or in an improperly tested drug; and in using community facilities in the total care of chronic illness. A firm link between the hospital and the health department can best be forged by having both under the same administrator. The cities of New York and Boston are already experimenting with such a plan.

Voluntary Health Agencies

Provision also must be made to bring voluntary health agencies within the functional scope of the hospital center. Those providing direct services — for example, the visiting nurse association — must be housed within the center. If the visiting nurse is to act under the supervision of the physician in establishing liaison between home and hospital care, she must be close by.

With regard to the many voluntary health agencies not providing direct services, it is likely that society will eventually tire of the continuing wasteful proliferation of individual health agencies each devoted to a single disease or organ system. Some day there will evolve a single, strong voluntary organization in the hospital center to work directly with the local health department and to be composed of many subunits, each channeling the interest of its supporters toward the conquest of its own health problem.

Although regionalization of medical facilities may sound complicated and difficult, it is unreasonable to believe that it would not be more successful than our present chaotic, catch-as-catch-can lack of system that is so seriously in trouble. At least, we must begin with carefully designed studies, the application of operations research, the immediate sharing of services, and the elimination of duplication among institutions, facilities, and personnel in the area.

Medical Personnel

With the documented scarcity of all kinds of medical personnel, the complaints on every side of not being able to "find a doctor" or "get a nurse," it is essential that a plan for the future must contain proposals for their more efficient use.

The General Physician — In Limbo[6]

We have seen how the specialist has evolved to a well-established and secure future while the general practitioner remains in limbo. The rapid evolution of the medical care constellation with its ever more varied personnel and increasing complexity of structure makes it all the more necessary that one individual, possibly the general physician, be responsible for effective interaction within it, for the benefit of the patient. In principle, this new responsibility could be added to those already within

[6] The "general physician" as used here refers to the general practitioner in modern dress responsible for primary care, continuity of care, personal health services, and reassurance to the patient. Many other terms are currently in use, including family doctor, primary physician, and general practitioner. This term does not refer to the qualified internist or pediatrician.

the scope of the general physician, which include primary management, continuity of care, personal health services, and reassurance of his patients. But the number of general physicians is rapidly diminishing; they are not being replaced; and if the trend continues, in two or three decades they will have disappeared. What can be done about it? I do not honestly know exactly how these services are to be provided. This appears to be the most difficult of all the problems in the medicine of the future. There are a number of possibilities. Let us explore them.

We may continue to do nothing. We shall, of course, as at present, receive intermittent general health services when we are cared for by those specialists who make a conscious effort to meet this need. Some general internists and pediatricians will provide these services, but mostly for the relatively small proportion of our population living in upper-middle-class suburbs adjacent to our major cities. Others will have to turn to the emergency services of general hospitals in urban areas, to graduates of substandard foreign medical schools, to osteopaths, to the local druggist, to relatives and friends, to chiropractors or quacks, or treat themselves with patent medicines.

If physicians fail to provide general health services, another medical profession, such as public health nursing, may have to be upgraded to take on these responsibilities. If so, the public health nurses would not be too different from the Russian women physicians practicing in small dispensaries throughout that large nation. In some rural areas in the United States, public health nurses actually perform many of the duties that are usually the responsibility of the licensed general physician although theoretically they act only under his direction.

It has been suggested that there is no need for a person to perform these duties. Some believe that a program can be written so that automated equipment and a computer could provide general health services.[7] I do not share this feeling.

Among the many possibilities, I would still hope that a physician, a member of a group practice unit and affiliated with a regional medical care system, would be educated specifically for this task. But this cannot come to pass unless three conditions are satisfied. Society must clearly understand his role, demand his services, and be willing to compensate him accordingly. The hospital must appoint him on its staff and assign to him the responsibility for providing continuity of care for patients within and without its walls. Medical schools must modify their admission policies and their curricula to assure his matriculation and education.

But this may be wishful thinking. It is more likely that the services for which the general physician is responsible

[7] A number of engineers attending my lectures at the Massachusetts Institute of Technology expressed this point of view strongly. Michael Godfrey, a graduate student in the Department of Mechanical Engineering, proposed that what was really needed was a "warm computer."

will not be generally available and that various combinations of these possibilities will evolve and obtain in different localities. The future is cloudy, but because these tasks loom so large in the medical care of the future, this question deserves wide and enlightened public and professional discussion.

The Nurse of the Future

The wide range of duties and responsibilities now expected of the nurse clearly does not fit any single pattern of aptitude or education. As a result, it is simply impossible to relate the total responsibilities of all kinds of nurses to any single clear-cut educational program. The recent position paper of the American Nursing Association recommending college education for all nurses is therefore clearly unrealistic. To be sure, nurses with top-level responsibilities will need a college education. But, in general, the responsibilities now allocated to the "nurse" must be divided in accordance with the aptitude, background, education, and training needed to perform specific tasks. Only by a series of definitions of categories and by a careful analysis of tasks can the educational needs be defined. And when these decisions are made and implemented, each of the categories must have a new name. The word "nurse" cannot be used for all of them if the present confusion is to be eliminated.

For the same reasons, it is simply impossible to set up a single nursing fee schedule. There must be a separate fee schedule for each category of "nurse" in order that reimbursement be commensurate with the services provided.

With utter confusion in status, and with inadequate and often inappropriate pay schedules, it is no wonder that recruitment of nurses in the United States has been unsuccessful. If recruitment is to be effective, a realistic plan for the future cannot treat the nursing profession as a single unit. Our plan for the future must bring an end to the perpetual wrangling over the status of the nurse by looking with new eyes at the problem as a whole.

This nursing example outlines the process that must be followed for each of the medical professions and vocations. Using data collected with specific relevance to medical care needs, systems analysis should make possible a more efficient use of medical personnel in our complex system of medical care.

Need for a General Plan

We have seen how tasks not demanding the qualifications of a doctor or a nurse may be delegated to others with less education and experience, how the control of complex systems may interrelate their functions more effectively, and how automation and technology may take over special tasks and thereby save professional time. Now we must outline a plan to take all of these factors into consideration. The time released by increasing efficiency in these many different ways will, in effect, increase the total number of our physicians, nurses, and other members of the medical professions.

Assuming that we have identified those tasks of each of the health and medical professions that demand its competence, how are we to decide to whom the other tasks may be delegated? There are no studies in the civilian population of the United States of the total interlocking functions of medical, professional, and vocational personnel. There are, of course, models of limited programs in the civilian population. The Kaiser Permanente Program in California is an experiment with group practice in specially designed hospitals for insured populations. We should take advantage of such experience. But we shall have to look elsewhere for models of total medical care programs to determine how best to interrelate the functions of all medical personnel.

Fortunately, there are other models. The Armed Services, because of their peculiar needs for providing emergency medical care under field conditions and for giving up-to-date and fairly complete medical care to relatively small groups of geographically isolated personnel, have evolved systems in which specially trained nonmedical personnel have taken over many tasks performed in the civilian population by physicians, nurses, and members of other medical professions.

We have been examining the programs of the United States Army, Air Force, and Navy. Each has had valuable experience that we believe can be adapted to civilian needs. To be sure, military programs cannot be transferred directly to the civilian population. In the Armed Forces, the physician and the nurse not only have professional status but also carry the command authority of officers over enlisted corpsmen. Moreover, we can adapt to the civilian population only those features of the military program that are free of the authoritarianism implicit in the structure of the military services. Nevertheless, it should be possible to adapt for civilian use much of their experience in the delegation of medical duties to nonmedical personnel, without compromising the principles of a free and open democratic society.

The United States Navy, because of its special needs created by widespread deployment in relatively small units over the surface of the entire globe, has been forced to develop the most comprehensive medical care programs. The hospital corpsman at the beginning of his career performs simple tasks under close supervision in the station hospital. As he does these successfully, he undergoes additional training and is given gradually increasing responsibility. Eventually, he may be assigned to a destroyer to provide simple medical care and, when necessary, to perform more complicated medical procedures under orders sent to him by radio from a physician who may be hundreds or thousands of miles away.

Underlying this use of nonmedical personnel in the Navy is a carefully defined program. The basic educational qualifications for admission to the Hospital Corps of the Navy have been defined. High-school graduates can qualify for the first course by passing the basic aptitude tests. After passing the first course, the corpsman then begins his medical service in the station hospital. His progression up the scale depends on his ability, competence, and interest. The curricula of the required courses for each step along the way have been set. The order of progression from simple to more complicated and from general to more specialized tasks has been laid out. For each task, the amount of responsibility to be assigned to the corpsman has been decided and the degree and kind of medical and nursing supervision necessary for safe and effective medical care have been specified.

As in the case of most medical care programs, the precise effectiveness in terms of health and disease of the military medical programs is unknown. Its comparative effectiveness with civilian medical care has not yet been ascertained. Moreover, it cannot be decided *a priori* which aspects of the military programs can be applied to civilian medical care.

But one thing is clear. Certain medical tasks usually performed by physicians or nurses in the civilian population appear to be successfully carried out by supervised nonmedical personnel in the Armed Forces. These include specifically defined physical examinations, the treatment of minor illnesses and injuries, application of casts and traction following fractures, collection of blood for transfusion and/or analysis, intravenous treatment with blood and blood derivatives, the administration and supervision of drug treatments, and immunizing procedures. Most important of all in terms of adapting the medical program of the Armed Forces to civilian medical care is the participation of the medical corpsman in the care of civilian dependents of the Armed Forces.

The study of the medical programs of the Armed Forces for purposes of translation to civilian populations cannot be performed in random fashion by individual investigators nor by isolated groups of research workers. The investigators must have enough authority to work closely with the Department of Defense to evaluate the effectiveness of the military medical program in terms of health and disease. When the data are collected and interpreted, the results for civilian use must be acceptable to physicians and to members of the other medical professions and vocations. Model civilian programs as they are put into operation will have to be related to public expectations. Finances, staffing, and long-range continuity must be assured.

The military experience in medical care can probably be extended to the civilian population through one of two mechanisms: the National Advisory Council on Health Manpower could be converted into a permanent Presidential Commission with long-range authority to conduct research and recommend programs; or the National Academy of Sciences, through the Medical Division of the National Research Council, could extend its activities to include research on mechanisms for providing medical care.

Whatever the mechanisms, the physicians of our country will have a magnificent opportunity to demonstrate statesmanship in evaluating existing programs and in making recommendations for change to benefit the patient. One can only hope that the medical profession will supply the necessary leadership and not continue to permit major changes in medical practice to occur by default, as they did with Medicare.

There are civilian models covering limited and specific problems that must also be studied. In the face of our unsatisfactory infant mortality rates, it would be reasonable, for example, to study programs in those countries that do much better than we do. In every other Western country where infant mortality is lower than in the United States, there is a medically supervised nurse-midwifery system. Such systems will have to be carefully evaluated and adapted to practice in our country.

Changes in legislation will also be needed to bring the benefits of the new nurse-midwifery system to American mothers and their babies. At present, only two states, Kentucky and New Mexico, and the city of New York have licensure laws that permit the practice of nurse-midwifery under medical supervision. Indeed, throughout the implementation of the plan, state licensure and other laws would have to be amended to accommodate for the reallocation of medical tasks.

Technology and Automation

The accelerating trends interrelating technology and automation with medicine and biology can be projected into the future. When laboratory tests are automated, I, as a physician, should like to have on my desk every morning a "printout" from the computer of the tests I ordered on the previous day, with all of the abnormal results standing out in capital letters in red ink. Each test would be reported on a line, starting with the name of the patient, giving the result of the test, the range of normal for the patient (for example, age, sex), and ending with an interpretation of the results. Test results that have serious implications for the patient's well-being would be starred in bright red ink.

The computer would not only supply me with a reliable fool-proof checked laboratory report (and tell me to repeat the test if it were unsatisfactory) but could also provide the opportunity for continuous postgraduate education on the meaning of laboratory results in the prevention and treatment of disease. Going one step further, when the implications of a report were extremely serious for the patient, the computer could figuratively give me a friendly but urgent tap on the shoulder. After the appropriate number of days, it would "print out" a question asking me whether or not Mrs. Jones had responded well to the lifesaving treatment that I should have prescribed when I received the report of the abnormal findings of the test.

Similar kinds of projections can be made concerning the potential benefits of computer-controlled drug administration to eliminate human error, to assure effective drug treatment, and to provide up-to-date postgraduate education for the physician about drug therapy.

Medical Diagnosis in the Future

I have told you how our studies on the diagnosis of patients with pain in the chest led us to recommend, as a screening test, a chest film as the first step in the diagnosis of any patient with that chief complaint. A general principle became evident. A set of screening tests that are relevant to the patients' chief complaints could be defined to give the physician a point of departure toward a diagnosis. Thus, a patient with the chief complaint of jaundice, for example, now has his liver function measured by a battery of tests performed during his first few days in the hospital. In the future, the chief complaint of jaundice should set off a train of events upon entry to the hospital in which appropriate specimens would be collected and an automated battery of liver tests run off immediately so that the results would be available to the diagnosing physician.

Every chief complaint would have its particular battery of screening tests performed as soon as possible after arrival at the hospital so that the physician would have essential diagnostic information at hand when he "works up" his patient. Diagnosis would become a directed instead of a random process. Studies are now under way to relate chief complaints of patients to appropriate screening and diagnostic tests, which, if properly built into the admission procedure, should increase the rapidity and efficiency of diagnosis.

In essence this procedure is an example of how we may take advantage in medical care of modern automation and technology. It also has significant implications for the structure of our medical care system. The physician practicing alone without such modern aids will become an anachronism. Moreover, the efficient application of automation and technology to medicine lends further weight to the arguments for a regionalized medical care system in which the physician has his office in a group practice unit immediately accessible to the facilities and equipment of the hospital center.

There is another immediate application. Because of the urgent need for medical care for the residents of the slums of our large cities, the suggestion has been made that diagnosis and treatment centers be located within them. Unfortunately, this appealing suggestion is impractical because of the inaccessibility of technical facilities and the scarcity of medical personnel. It would make more sense to establish an ambulatory treatment center adjacent to the hospital, accessible to its equipment, services, and personnel, and linked to a small information and guidance center in the needy area by a transportation system. In the guidance center, appropriately trained public health nurses, who would also make home visits, would greet the patients, analyze their problems, and refer those requiring medical care to the ambulatory center by way of the transportation system and, if necessary, to the inpatient service of the hospital itself.

Retrieval of Medical Information

As I have stated elsewhere,[8] automation and technology could be useful in helping physicians to maintain contact with medical knowledge and in guiding research workers to retrieve information from the medical literature. But an automated system by itself is not enough. "Medlars," the medical retrieval system currently used in this country which selects a scientific report by key words in the title or text, is proving to be unsatisfactory because it retrieves too many inappropriate articles. In effect, it forces the investigator to read each article selected by the system to find out if he needs to read it for his research purposes.

A retrieval system, to provide a research worker with

[8] David D. Rutstein, "Maintaining Contact with Medical Knowledge," Presidential address to the Sesquicentennial of the Boylston Medical Society, Boston, Mass., May 25, 1961.

a list of more appropriate articles, demands evaluation and coding of each article by an expert in the field. A simple system, in which the referee for the medical journal would code each article recommended for publication, should satisfy this need.

Similarly, automated retrieval could help the practicing physician to keep up to date. But, again, the system alone will not suffice. It must be bolstered by an organized series of review articles. Here we may learn much from the legal profession. The law is based on precedent. Every lawyer must be able to find out whether "someone else got away with it before." Moreover, every judicial decision is a review article. In the late nineteenth century when Justice Louis Brandeis was on the faculty of the Harvard Law School, he stimulated the law students to integrate judicial decisions covering a particular legal point into review articles, and the Harvard Law Review was born. We need exactly the same kind of critical review articles in medicine so that the practicing physician may quickly get the "last word" to his patient. Indeed, we need a "Harvard Medical Review" and many other university medical reviews, bolstered by a system for automated retrieval of medical knowledge.

Research in the Future

Research to yield fundamental knowledge in biological and medical systems must be continued, strengthened, and expanded. Such knowledge is the foundation for all of our efforts in improving health and in the prevention and treatment of disease. Indeed, laboratory research during the past few decades has been the rock upon which much of our progress has been based. Knowledge discovered with the guidance of the scientific method is the key to the solution of our pressing medical problems. But, as we have already seen, the contributions of technology, automation, and the computer make it possible to design studies and to discover knowledge in more complex systems so that the knowledge revealed may be of more immediate importance to human health.

To take advantage of this new approach, we must modify what has become the snobbish attitude of the laboratory investigator to the clinical research worker. This attitude has undoubtedly influenced the allocation of available medical research funds, which in turn has reinforced the attitude. We need a better balance in our medical research program. There is so much talk about "basic research," usually undefined. Sometimes when I hear this repeated over and over it sounds as if the speaker were saying, "basic research is the research that *I* do."

As a result, the reputation of clinical investigation has suffered unjustifiably, and the clinical research worker has tended to renounce his field for the more orthodox occupation of the laboratory investigator. If we remember that science is a method of reasoning and not a function of the complexity of the laboratory equipment used in a study, we see that it is equally applicable to the laboratory and to the clinic. Clinical investigation *has* yielded facts upon which general biological laws are based. For instance, the discovery of vaccination against smallpox by Jenner in the 1790's led to the general principles of immunization.

To be sure, the rigorous application of the scientific method to clinical investigation is very difficult. But it is a real challenge to use our new tools and to design studies that might yield results immediately applicable to man. In urging this, I want to make it clear that there is no conflict between the rigorous application of the scientific method in ethical clinical investigation and the spirit of dedication of the physician to his patient. Since knowledge of health and disease in man is fundamental to the relief of human suffering, let us not continue to emulate the intoxicated gentleman who late one night was crawling on his hands and knees under a street light looking for his wallet. "Did you lose it here?" asked a passer-by. "No," said the drunk, pointing off in the direction of the other side of the street, "but it's dark over there."

Let us not be misled. The discovery of knowledge about health and disease in man will not in itself make its benefits available. To do this, we also need precise knowledge about the factors that affect the delivery of medical care. We have so little knowledge about that problem. Fortunately, operations research, so successful in war games and industry, is now, as I have pointed out, being applied to the field of health. But, such application presupposes sound and precise data. If the theoretical knowledge of the mechanisms for the control of complex systems is to be applied to medical care, we must first develop research programs to reveal knowledge of the same high quality as that being discovered in biological systems. Community health research centers, in which rigorous scientific investigation will yield the kind and quality of information required for precise planning, are urgently needed.

We can also look forward to a new dimension in the study of biological systems and of systems of medical care when they are buttressed by the disciplines of mathematics, the physical and engineering sciences, and technology. We do have the great responsibility of unifying our efforts for human betterment.

Medical Curriculum

There is international disquietude about the status and validity of the curriculum to which our medical students are now being exposed. During the past year, I had the privilege of attending meetings of the Swedish Medical Curriculum Committee at Uppsala and the Committee on Undergraduate Education of the Royal Commission on Medical Education in London. Members of American medical faculties constantly bring up the subject, and the Harvard medical faculty is now paying more attention to the medical curriculum than to any other single matter. As one goes from one meeting to the next, the problems raised seem always to be the same.

The changing role of the physician in medical care and research underlies much of the anxiety that has precipitated this sudden spate of interest in the medical curriculum. And yet, curiously enough, little effort is being made to relate curricular planning to a projection of the physician's future role. In this proposal I shall attempt to do so. Indeed, the contents of these lectures provide the guidelines to a projection of that role and the background against which the following curricular plan is to be viewed.

Obvious at once is the discrepancy between the widening spectrum of career opportunities in medicine, and of the background of matriculating medical students, and the narrow, rigid medical curriculum.

The range of career opportunities is constantly being added to as medicine becomes ever more complex. In recent years we have seen the appearance of new medical careers such as those of specialists in the fields of artificial organs, in organ transplantation, in open-heart surgery, and in clinical preventive medicine, experts in international medical care and biomathematics, to name a few.

At the other extreme we see a major change in the composition of entering medical school classes. Until a decade ago, at the Harvard Medical School most students matriculated with a standard premedical education in the biomedical sciences and with a smattering of physics and mathematics. A few students concentrated in the humanities and in the social sciences and took a minimum of premedical laboratory science.

Later, we began to see a trend away from organic chemistry toward biology. And during the past few years there has been a marked shift toward mathematics, physics, and engineering. Indeed, about one fifth of the matriculating class at the Harvard Medical School in 1967 will have concentrated their college education in these three areas.[9] Medical school classes are becoming more heterogeneous, and the small annual moves and occasional jumps in the medical curriculum checker games do not take these radical changes in the structure of the student body into account.

Medical faculties are beginning to recognize more and more that with the explosion of medical knowledge and increasing specialization there must be concomitantly an increasingly flexible medical curriculum. Indeed, it is becoming fashionable to speak about adding flexibility by designing a "core curriculum" and supplementing it with elective courses. The core curriculum would include all the essential teaching for all medical students. The core is to be surrounded by a large number of elective courses among which the students may pick and choose.

Unfortunately, the model does not meet the need. It is literally impossible to select *a priori* the core knowl-

[9] Daniel H. Funkenstein, "Data on the Preparation of Harvard Medical Students," forthcoming.

edge essential for all medical students without first defining a series of courses of study to take into account the background, education, motivation, aptitudes, and career objectives of each student. Moreover, any attempt to define an arbitrary core always favors the existing orthodoxy in the medical faculty and tends to stifle educational progress.

The projected elective program is also chaotic. The student, with the guidance of a faculty advisor, has to choose an appropriate curriculum from literally hundreds of elective courses in a large catalogue. In this system, the faculty abdicates its responsibility to the student for assembling a logical educational experience in a series of courses of study.

How, then, can we tailor the medical curriculum to meet the needs of the individual student? We do have a precedent. The evolution of the medical school curriculum is closely repeating the history of the curriculum in the college.

At Harvard College, from 1642 to 1825, when the primary objective was the education of young men for the ministry, candidates for the Bachelor's Degree had a fixed curriculum. With the reforms proposed by Professor George Ticknor, elective courses were introduced. During the last half of the nineteenth century, President Charles W. Eliot developed a perhaps too flexible elective system. Within it, students could pick their way through the four years of college earning their gentleman's C's in the less demanding courses. Clearly, reform was once again necessary. The college faculty under the guidance of President A. Lawrence Lowell reasserted its authority in the early twentieth century and accepted responsibility for defining requirements and the flexibility of the curriculum.

The curriculum at Harvard College now consists of a combination of required and elective courses: the student concentrates in one area and distributes his other courses in accordance with a set of rules approved by the faculty. This set of faculty rules supplemented by departmental requirements establishes a range of patterns to guide the student in the selection and order of his courses toward a defined goal and a wide range of interests. Moreover, if the student changes his mind in midstream he is permitted to take additional courses and to start off in his new direction. With such a curriculum, Harvard College now educates young men for all of the professions and for many other callings.

If the Medical School curriculum followed the present Harvard College pattern it could meet the students' needs. Alternative courses of study, each for a defined medical career, when established by the faculty would provide appropriate preclinical and clinical education. As in the Harvard College pattern, each individual course of study would not be rigid but would offer a variety of elective choices. When all of the courses of study are laid out, their common curricular content would automatically define the actual core curriculum and obviate the need for *a priori* decisions.

But how will each department establish a series of channels at each stage along the way to provide the necessary flexibility? One answer is suggested by an educational experiment we have been conducting in the Department of Preventive Medicine.

In the 1950's, the course we offered in biostatistics — the rules by which things are counted in biological systems — was a constant source of discomfort to the students. It was far from a success. The spectrum of the students' mathematical abilities was wide — extending all the way from a bare understanding of algebra to a competent knowledge of mathematics. The usual course in biostatistics was aimed at the center of this range. The result was chaotic. A large segment of the class complained of the mathematical difficulty of the course, while a sizable group at the other extreme scorned it because for them it was trivial.

During the late 1950's a collaborative program in mathematics and medicine was developed between the Research Laboratory of Electronics at the Massachusetts Institute of Technology and the Department of Preventive Medicine at the Harvard Medical School. A biomathematician at the Massachusetts Institute of Technology — Professor Murray Eden — was appointed a Visiting Lecturer at the Harvard Medical School. This development occurred at a favorable moment, because it was already becoming clear that a single, rigid medical curriculum could no longer meet the needs of modern medicine. The collaboration of a biomathematician within the Department and the unsatisfactory state of biostatistical teaching provided an unusual opportunity to experiment with a double-channel course. The students were given the option of taking the standard course in biostatistics or qualifying for a course in the application of mathematical theory to biology and medicine. Those choosing the second option were given a manual, a set of problems, and a consultant instructor. If they passed the qualifying examination with an honor grade they were admitted to the course in biomathematics.

How did it work? It worked well and it worked badly. The biostatistics course now more closely fitted the spectrum of the class and was highly successful. The biomathematics course, however, proved to be unsatisfactory. Again, there was too wide a range of ability — there were no more than about a dozen students who were qualified in mathematics but about thirty students who could pass the qualifying examination.

After several years of experimentation, the solution became obvious. We needed a triple-channeled curriculum — a basic course in biostatistics focused on the intelligent reading of the medical literature for the future practicing physician; an intermediate course in biostatistics concerned with the design of medical experiments for the future research physician; and a demanding course in the application of mathematical theory to medicine and biology (just as it has been applied to physics during the past half century) for the gifted, highly motivated mathematical student.

This triple-channeled curriculum has been successful in many ways. It is now tailored to fit the student's background, ability, education, motivations, and career objectives. It also offers the gifted student the unusual opportunity of becoming conversant with a new medical field, and he does not waste his time taking a course that he could master by himself.

This experiment establishes a model upon which a flexible medical curriculum could be based. If each department would offer a planned series of choices to the students, the permutations and combinations of channels would truly make it possible to tailor the entire curriculum to meet the needs of the individual student. It also exposes the student to every discipline so that, notwithstanding his future career objectives, he would become aware of the relation of his field of interest to all of medicine. Such a *horizontally expanded* curriculum helps each student to progress at a maximum rate without increasing the length of the total curriculum. Moreover, it permits the student to follow his own bent.

The proposed medical curriculum takes into account the principles of concentration and distribution of the college curriculum. The student can both advance in the field of his own interest and become aware of the potential contributions of the other medical specialties.

The proposed curriculum would allow for the inclusion of different disciplines as they become relevant to medicine and biology. The disciplines at the Massachusetts Institute of Technology are good examples. The physicist could contribute fluid dynamic theory to teaching about the circulation of the blood; the engineer, his design of an electronic prosthesis to the instruction in orthopedics; the mathematician, his model of the equilibrium between gas and liquid to the exploration of lung function; and the computer specialist, his methods for simulating the function of the human kidney or the complex operation of a hospital. Finally, the proposed curriculum could be broad enough to accommodate the entire range of future medical careers from the general physician to the bio-mathematician.

We have presented in broad outline one plan for the medicine of the future. It matters not whether this particular plan is followed, but it is essential that an effective plan be developed, and quickly. Such development presupposes an intensive research program to guide the evolution of the plan.

Whatever the plan, it must resolve the paradox of modern medicine, direct the inevitable pressures in a constructive way, interrelate the effective practice of the physician and of all other medical personnel, allow for the analysis and control of complex institutional systems, take advantage of the growing opportunities in automation and technology in the improvement of medical care and for more effective design of experiments in biological and medical research, and educate the medical student not for the present but for the medicine of the future.

Appendix

Evidence has been accumulated during the past twenty years in the Department of Preventive Medicine at the Harvard Medical School that realistic and comprehensive standards of medical care can be established. Every year since 1947 each student in the fourth-year class has performed a Health Resources Survey of a community, in which optimal standards for care are defined. Since the details of the survey procedure may be useful in future attempts to set medical standards, the actual instructions given to the students are supplied in this appendix.

Harvard Medical School

Department of Preventive Medicine

*Instructions for Performance
of Health Resources Survey — 1966*

Up to this time you have been learning to become a physician in a medical school and in teaching hospitals where more and better resources exist for the care of patients than you are likely to find in the average community. The principal objectives of this survey are to make you more aware of your responsibility to provide the highest quality of medical care possible for your patients under the conditions existing in your community and to encourage you to consider practical means for improvement. We expect you to demonstrate an adequate awareness and thorough understanding of community health resources, since these are essential for the practice of good medicine.

A brief medical history and pertinent physical findings in each of four cases are attached, along with information about socioeconomic status. You are to prepare a detailed statement of the diagnostic, therapeutic, and *preventive resources* that you would require for the optimal management of each patient. These should not be limited to the obvious ones provided by a physician in a general hospital but should include all those institutional and community resources that might be used to improve the status of the patient. Thus, a patient suffering from tuberculosis might require the services of a general physician, a specialist, public health nurse, medical social worker, occupational therapist, special hospital or facilities for convalescent care, and perhaps vocational guidance. Preventive services are to be outlined from the point of view of preventing spread of disease to others, complications, and disability in or death of the patient. In addition, discuss in each case measures that might have been of some help if they had been instituted prior to the development of disease.

Following the preparation of the statement of optimal resources, you are to go to a community of your choice to collect and record data about the personnel, organizations, and services that actually exist for the complete management of the four cases. In each case assume that *you are the responsible physician* and indicate how you would make the best use of the available resources. It is expected that you will show evidence of a thorough understanding of the type, quality, and scope of the required services as well as the means for their implementation. In general, the two most useful methods for obtaining information about the medical assets of a community are (1) personal interviews with physicians, hospital administrators, public health officers, and other representatives of governmental and voluntary agencies in the health and welfare field, and (2) reference to published material such as that dealing with the qualifications and number of physicians, classification and description of hospitals, medical care plans, and welfare agencies. It is desirable to use more than one source of information in your evaluation, since a critical appraisal of the quality of medical care cannot be accomplished without comparisons of facts and opinions. Document the sources of information by listing the names of all individuals or agency representatives interviewed. You are not required to prepare a complete analysis of all community health assets, but rather you are expected to find the *best channel of care for your patients* in view of the most probable diagnosis in each case.

Finally, you are to compare the conditions existing in the community with your statement of optimal resources and write a critical discussion of the differences. It is expected that you will relate your recommendations to existing community agencies or those that might be developed. You should not recommend an unattainable Utopian solution.

An introductory section should provide a general description of the community and its resources, with reference made to those personnel, agencies, and services to be used in the management of the four cases. Then each case should be presented as a unit, clearly indicating the specific application of the resources to each patient. Your recommendations should be numbered so that they may be readily identified by the reader.

Thus, your survey report will include:

1. Introduction
2. Optimal resources
3. Actual resources
4. Differences and recommendations
5. Documentation of sources of information and interviews

Following the submission and evaluation of your report, arrangements will be made for a conference between you and a faculty member to discuss the survey.

CASE 1

You are called to the hospital on a Saturday afternoon to see a 3½-year-old boy who is brought to the hospital by his father. The father, who is separated from his wife, became alarmed by his son's condition when he visited his wife and three children a short time earlier. According to the mother the child had eaten very little for about three days and had vomited greenish-brown material immediately after eating.

The patient had several admissions to another hospital. A report from that hospital indicated that during the second month of life he was admitted with "convulsions." He was found to have a nondepressed parietal skull fracture with subdural effusion. Two months later, at the age of five months, he was readmitted with a recurrent subdural effusion, which was again tapped. At about one year of age he was again admitted with a dislocated shoulder.

Four weeks prior to the present admission the child was brought to the emergency room with multiple ecchymoses of the head, face, chest, abdomen, and extremities. A week later on examination the ecchymoses were noted to be clearing. A third appointment was broken.

A review of systems revealed that the patient's head has always seemed large. According to the mother the child's personality has changed recently, he has become unresponsive to commands, and he has slapped his mother.

On physical examination on this admission the child measured 37½″ in length and weighed 24 pounds. The blood pressure was 120/60, pulse 120, respiration 20. The child appeared acutely ill, was somewhat unresponsive and withdrawn, and moved only his extremities. Contusions were seen on the face, the scalp, on the right ear, the penis, over the anterior surface of the left tibia. There was a large bruise in the suprapubic region. Skin turgor was decreased. The throat and mouth were dry. Abdomen was protuberant, somewhat tympanitic, and had a "doughy" quality. Generalized tenderness was noted on palpation with questionable rebound tenderness. There were no bowel sounds. There was suprapubic dullness and dullness in the right lower quadrant. Neurological examination revealed intact sensation and intact, although weak, motor function.

Laboratory Data: Admission hematocrit was 38 per cent and the white count 3500. Urinalysis showed a specific gravity of 1.025, a trace of albumin, and an occasional white cell. Electrolytes were: Na 128, K 4.0, Cl 86. Chest film was unremarkable. X rays demonstrated gross distension of the small bowel and extensive collection of fluid in the peritoneal cavity. There was no gas in the colon. The picture was consistent with paralytic ileus.

A surgical consultant decided that immediate surgery was necessary. At operation a perforated distal ileum was found. The perforated ileum was resected and end-to-end anastomosis performed. The surgeon found extensive peritoneal exudate which he felt must have been present for some days. Postoperatively the patient had a stormy course with intermittent small bowel obstruction, which was treated by Miller-Abbot tube drainage. By the fourth postoperative week the child was beginning to take fluids by mouth and was much improved.

In addition, pampering by the nursing staff began to produce a change in the child's personality. He became less withdrawn and more communicative. He nevertheless continued to have temper tantrums at times and was felt to be a continuing psychological problem. During the last week of hospitalization the patient was noted to play with other children, nurses, doctors, and to improve in attitude and in interest in the world around him.

Social History: The father and mother are separated. On the Saturday afternoon when the boy was first brought to the hospital the father, while visiting his family, had observed the bruises found at admission. Because he suspected that the mother had mistreated the child and because of the child's obvious illness, he immediately brought him to the hospital.

The patient's father is age 29 and is a house painter. The mother is 19 years of age and is presently under psychiatric care. The father informs you that their marriage has been a stormy one with violent quarrels, with repeated separations and reconciliations. He seems to be quite immature.

There are two children in the family in addition to the patient. Their ages are two years and one year. Their development has apparently been normal and they have not had any unusual illnesses.

When you asked the mother to come in and see you

she broke her first appointment but kept the second one. She appeared to lack affection and appropriate concern for the child. She had explanations for everything that had happened to the child, which were often volunteered before she was asked about specific events. She stated that she was unable to cope with the child's tantrums. She felt that the child was mentally subnormal. The mother does not know the whereabouts of her parents. The patient's father lives most of the time with his parents. The paternal grandfather is a laboring man who owns a modest home in a working-class neighborhood. The paternal grandmother seems to be a sensible lady of about 60 years who visited her grandson several times during his hospital stay.

CASE 2

You are called by a pediatrician who asks if you will see Mrs. K. without delay. The pediatrician is taking care of her two-month old son on whom he has made a tentative diagnosis of tuberculosis meningitis.

When Mrs. K. comes to your office she looks very well. Her age is 41 years. Upon questioning it develops that she has a slight cough productive of a small amount of white sputum but she denies having any recent illness or any incapacity. She has not had any fever, any unusual weight loss, night sweats, or fatigue. Indeed, she states that she has a great deal of energy. For the past four or five years she has slept only four or five hours each night and never goes to bed until about 2:00 A.M. On persistent questioning, she recalls that she had an episode of pleurisy that lasted about two weeks fifteen years previously.

Physical examination: T:99, P:126, BP:118/74. There was marked resonance of the upper half of her right lung. There was complete absence of breath sounds in this area with some suggestion of distant amphoric breathing; numerous crackles were heard over the right lung base posteriorly. The left lung was clear throughout. Her hemoglobin was 10 grams, WBC, 14,500 with 75 per cent polys. The sputum showed many acid-fast bacilli, and a first strength PPD subsequently showed 10 millimeters of induration. Sputum culture that was taken at the first visit subsequently showed acid-fast bacilli identified as human tubercle bacilli.

The chest X ray revealed a large area of radiolucency in the upper half of the right lung that is interpreted as either a large cavity or a localized pneumothorax. The lung immediately below this shows infiltration consistent with tuberculosis.

The patient has been married for twelve years. Although she and her husband have wanted several children, her two-month old baby represents the only pregnancy that has been carried to term. Six years previously she was admitted to a university hospital for D & C and investigation relative to sterility. At that time a routine chest X ray was taken and the responsible doctor informed her that she had a small spot on her lung "about which she did not need to be concerned." The radiologist at the university hospital reported that the film taken six years previously showed a cavity in the RUL. She did not have either an X ray or a PPD in the course of her recent successful pregnancy.

The pediatrician later reports that the baby's meningitis was proved to be tuberculosis by smear of the pellicle and culture of the CSF.

The husband, upon investigation, is found to have a positive first strength PPD but no other evidence of tuberculosis.

Mr. K is a self-employed consulting engineer who travels extensively in carrying out his business. His net income is usually between $15,000 and $20,000 per year. He carries a commercial hospital insurance policy that guarantees him $15.00 for each day of hospitalization. In addition, he has major medical insurance, which reimburses him for 80 per cent of all expenditures between $500 and $10,000 in each episode of illness. His spouse is covered by this policy but he has done nothing to assure the child's inclusion so is unsure about whether the son is covered. Mrs. K had worked as an executive secretary in a local office until the second month of her recent pregnancy. In the course of her work she supervised several young clerical workers and, in handling the payroll for some forty workers, came into contact with most of the concern's local employees.

Case 3

Shortly after the death of your senior partner, you are asked to see one of his patients.

Mr. M is a 43-year-old minor executive in a chain store organization. He comes to you at this time because he has been discharged from his job with the explanation that "his inability to get about" was interfering with his work.

The history of the present illness goes back fifteen years. At age 28, while playing tennis, Mr. M became aware that he often missed the ball, an unusual occurrence for him. He found that he finally had to abandon the game. A few months later he had an episode of double vision, which lasted about one month. He was well again until twelve years ago when he had an episode during which he was unable to walk and remained paralyzed for several days. There was gradual recovery thereafter. He was again entirely well until nine years ago when he discovered he was having difficulty walking and had a feeling as if there were "cushions under both feet."

Gradually increasing difficulty with walking has occurred since. One year ago the patient's balance became so impaired that he was no longer able to walk and was required to remain in a wheelchair. He has had urinary urgency, frequency, and incontinence. Urinary disturbance is sufficiently marked so that he requires a leg urinal when outside the house.

In the past year or two there has been some deterioration in mentation and loss of memory.

On examination the right optic disc was pathologically pale, there was nystagmus of the abducting eye on gaze in either direction, the reflexes were hyperactive below the waist; the plantars were both extensor. There was marked abnormality on finger-to-nose bilaterally. The patient was unable to stand without assistance. Position sense was diminished at the toes, vibratory sense was absent at the toes, ankles, knees, and iliac crests. Sensation to pin prick was intact.

The patient is married and has three children, one a sophomore at Princeton, the second a high school sophomore, the third in the third grade. He owns a house for which he paid $20,000 five years ago, which has a $12,000 mortgage. His medical insurance lapsed when he was discharged from his job six months previously. The patient has $4,000 in savings earmarked for the university education of his children. Mrs. M has had no significant occupational experience except as a housewife.

CASE 4

One gray day in February, just after a freezing rain, you are called by one of your patients, a 75-year-old retired printing press operator who, crying, tells you that his wife has just fallen and is unable to rise. Examination a short time later confirms your suspicion that she has fractured the neck of her femur.

The wife, age 72, has been under your care for obesity and arthritis. She is just a shade over five feet tall and weighs 225 pounds. Many attempts to induce her to lose weight have failed. It is clear that her degenerative arthritis, which is found mainly in her knees, is aggravated by her weight problem. She seems unable to remain on a diet. Food, she has told you, is her only pleasure and she cannot resist eating according to her whims.

The husband has moderately severe Parkinson's disease. Recently he has often been anxious, depressed, and fearful. His facial expression is typically masklike, his limbs are stiff, and he exhibits the festinating gait of persons with the disease. He also has some arthritis of his shoulders, back, and knees. He is slim, in contrast to his wife.

The couple derives support from Social Security pensions and somewhat irregular and small contributions from their only son, who lives in another city. They receive a small supplement from the Welfare Department to help them to pay rent on their house, which is located in a run-down neighborhood far from shopping facilities, churches, and recreation. The husband occasionally obtains a ride to the shopping center with neighbors, but his travel to and from community facilities is always a problem to him.

Contrast the problem of obtaining care for this patient (or couple) before and after implementation of the Medicare program (that is, before July 1, 1966, and after January 1, 1967).

Index